# Prescribing in General Practice

Edited by

CONRAD HARRIS

Prescribing Research Unit
University of Leeds

Foreword by

JANE RICHARDS

General Practitioner
Exeter

RADCLIFFE MEDICAL PRESS
OXFORD and NEW YORK

© 1996 Conrad Harris

Radcliffe Medical Press Ltd
18 Marcham Road, Abingdon, Oxon OX14 1AA, UK

Radcliffe Medical Press, Inc.
141 Fifth Avenue, New York, NY 10010, USA

British Library Cataloguing in Publication Data

A catalogue record for this book is available from the British Library.

ISBN 1 85775 042 X

Library of Congress Cataloging-in-Publication Data

Prescribing in general practice/edited by Conrad M. Harris.
   p. cm.
 Includes bibliographical references and index.
 ISBN 1-85775-042-X
 1. Drugs–Prescribing.   2. Family medicine.   I. Harris, Conrad M.
   (Conrad Michael)
   [DNLM: 1. Pharmacology, Clinical.   2. Pharmacokinetics.   3. Family Practice.
   QV 38 P933 1995]
   RM138.P72   1995
   615'.1–dc20
   DNLM/DLC
   for Library of Congress   95-33379
                                                                                    CIP

Typeset by Marksbury Typesetting, Midsomer Norton, Avon.
Printed and bound by Biddles Ltd, Guildford and King's Lynn.

Contents

The Business Side of General Practice
Editorial Board Members

List of contributors

Sir Michael Drury, OBE, FRCP, FRCGP, FRACGP, *Emeritus Professor of General Practice, University of Birmingham*

Rhiannon T Edwards, BSc (Econ) MA, *Lecturer in Health Economics, Department of Public Health Medicine, University of Liverpool*

Morgan P Feely, MD, FRCPI, *Senior Lecturer in Clinical Pharmacology, University of Leeds*

Peter R Fellows, MB, BS, *General Practitioner, Member of Prescribing Subcommittee GMSC and Advisory Committee on NHS Drugs*

John J Ferguson, TD, BSc, FRCGP, MICGP, MIBiol, MFFP, MHSM, *Medical Director, Prescription Pricing Authority, Newcastle-upon-Tyne*

Ravi S Gidar, BSc (Hons), Postgrad Dip Com Pharm, MRPharmS, *Community Pharmacist and Pharmaceutical Adviser, Ealing, Hammersmith & Hounslow Health Agency*

Conrad M Harris, M Ed, FRCGP, DRCOG, *Professor of General Practice, Director of the Prescribing Research Unit, University of Leeds; and General Practitioner*

Nicholas W Hough, BPharm, MSc, MRPharmS, *Director of Medicines Resource Centre (MeReC), Liverpool*

Jacqueline V Jolleys, BA, MBA, MD, MRCGP, *Honorary Lecturer in General Practice, University of Nottingham*

David E Pickersgill, MB, ChB, DObstRCOG, *General Practitioner, North Walsham, Norfolk*

Anne B Prasad, FRPharmS, *Executive Editor, BNF*

Philip M Reilly, MD, FRCGP, *Professor of General Practice, Queen's University of Belfast; and General Practitioner*

David J D Sleator, MB, BCh, BAO, BA, *Primary Care Development Directorate, West Surrey Health Commission*

Tom Walley, MD FRCPI, *Professor of Clinical Pharmacology, University of Liverpool*

Arnold Zermansky, MB, ChB, MRCGP, DObstRCOG, *General Practitioner, Honorary Senior Research Fellow, Department of General Practice, University of Leeds*

Jane Perekrest, BA, *Secretary to the Prescribing Research Unit. Her contribution is now invisible, but it was irreplaceable*

Foreword

Prescribing has been at the very core of general practice since an Act of 1542, the so-called 'Quack's Charter', permitted our forebears the apothecaries to supply simple herbal medicines to patients legally.

Today many more drug treatments are available; they are more powerful and thus potentially more dangerous and much more costly but the role of the general practitioner remains at the core of the prescribing process. Good prescribing should be rational and cost-effective and the chapters in this book cover many features of this complex subject which enable general practitioners to navigate between the rocks of temptations and the pools of patient needs. They signpost sources of information both printed and personal and discuss many contemporary concerns.

Do not be reticent about referring to it, even in front of patients, as it contains facts not easily found elsewhere. Read a chapter at a time or the whole book at once. Medicines and their prescribing are evolving all the time and I look forward to further editions of this book to mirror that evolution.

I know of no other single volume which includes as many of the important aspects of prescribing between two covers and I commend it to all my colleagues.

Jane Richards
General Practitioner,
Exeter and Chairman
of the Representative
Body British Medical
Association
October 1995

Introduction

The central dilemma of prescribing in general practice is easy to state. On the one hand, every prescription is an experiment; on the other, each general practitioner prescribes, on average, about 18 000 items a year. While working on this massive scale, we somehow have to cope with the need for a knowledge of hundreds of drugs, thousands of patients and a host of regulations, with the demands implicit in a scientific experimental approach – and we have to do so at the lowest possible expense.

No one can achieve this perfectly all the time, yet we are accountable for doing so. We need all the help we can get. The likelihood that many of our patients will recover regardless of what we do, together with a degree of good luck, probably plays a larger part in keeping us out of trouble than we may care to admit. For the rest, damage limitation would seem to be the best strategy. The less we prescribe, the less damage there will be to limit, but there still remains a formidable array of knowledge and skills that we have to master.

This book is intended as another source of help. It is a collection of chapters commissioned from experts, all but six of whom are, or have been, general practitioners. The chapters cover a wide range of topics; they are written in a variety of styles; and they bring together a rich spread of facts, regulations, ideas and opinions. They should be of interest to all general practitioners, from registrars to the most experienced. They are for browsing and also for consulting over practical matters; and in some cases they will be a useful source of reference.

This is not intended as a textbook, and it makes no claim to be comprehensive. As new issues arise, I hope they will find their way into the next edition along with additional topics that readers may request by writing to the publishers. Some aspects of prescribing are already so well covered in the *British National Formulary* (BNF) that there seemed no need to include them: prescription writing, including computer-issued prescriptions; the emergency supply of prescription-only medicines; prescribing for children and for the elderly; and prescribing in terminal care. The *BNF* is a mine of information on these and other matters that we all probably underuse.

Prescribing in General Practice is not like any other book on the market. I believe it will earn itself a place in every practice library and that it will benefit every general practitioner who writes prescriptions.

Conrad M Harris
November 1995

1 The basics of clinical pharmacology

Tom Walley

Many doctors have only vague ideas of what clinical pharmacology is and only distant memories of what they were taught about it. Clinical pharmacology is best defined as the study of drugs and their effects in people and on society. It clearly has an educational role for health care professionals and roles in drug development and drug safety. It also is very practical, addressing the optimal use of drug therapy for patient benefit while minimizing adverse effects. Some doctors argue that one does not need to know any clinical pharmacology to use drugs perfectly adequately. While this may work where prescribing is purely a reflex action, doctors today need to understand the basics of clinical pharmacology to make best use of existing drugs, especially in patients with complex problems, and to evaluate the many new drugs which emerge every year.

We will consider some basic principles of clinical pharmacology, and then move on to examine what drugs do to the body and what the body does to drugs.

Basic principles of clinical pharmacology

An American group defined what it called a core curriculum in clinical pharmacology for medical students. This included a number of items of essential knowledge, and certain skills and attitudes. While some of these are not really appropriate for British prescribers, many others state the basic principles of good drug use and are worth repeating here now, in a paraphrased form. Many of these are considered again later in this book. Mastering them can be achieved only by experience and personal reflection.

Knowledge

1 Basic pharmacokinetics applied to clinical situations – covered later in this chapter.

2 How to recognize and avoid adverse drug reactions, and what to do once you have recognized one; drug interactions – covered in Chapter 2.

3   Prescribing for special groups such as the elderly, the young, pregnant and breast-feeding women, and patients with kidney or liver disease – covered in the *British National Formulary*.

4   How to manage common drug overdoses, and a basic knowledge of drugs of abuse.

5   Regulations affecting prescribing – covered in several other chapters.

6   How drugs are developed and tested – covered in Chapter 15.

7   Criteria for selecting drugs for a personal formulary – covered in Chapter 9.

Skills and attitudes

8   How to learn about new drugs – covered in Chapter 17.

9   How to communicate and negotiate a therapeutic contract with the patient.

10   How to deal with the pressures to prescribe irrationally including: lack of time, patient and peer pressure, lack of knowledge, the pharmaceutical industry and advertising, and over-reliance on personal experience rather than evidence.

11   To understand that every prescription is an experiment, which may prove efficacious, toxic or both; the doctor must always weigh risks against benefits. Every prescription is written for an individual patient and there is no room for a 'cookbook' approach to prescribing.

12   To understand that rational prescribing must follow rational assessment of the patient, including diagnosis and investigation. This may be difficult in general practice because of the nature of early disease, and lack of time and resources for investigation: the GP often has to treat his best formulation of a patient's problem rather than a firm diagnosis, but should keep an open mind for clues which would change his formulation later.

13   To avoid both therapeutic paralysis and nihilism, whereby a doctor may be too concerned about the hazards of drugs to prescribe, and therapeutic adventurism, whereby he may not consider the adverse effects of a drug adequately in his enthusiasm to treat patients. This is particularly true in relation to the use of new drugs, which are not well studied before marketing and for which the true therapeutic role and the adverse effects only become clear with experience. Doctors should, therefore, be

conservative in their selection of drugs, and generally stick to the tried and tested, but not become fossilized and refuse wholesale to consider new drugs.

What drugs do to the body

This is called pharmacodynamics. The starting point is to consider how drugs work. Often we do not have a clear idea, and the proposed mechanism is a best guess which fits most of the observed facts. Many drugs act at receptors on target cell membranes and either activate the receptor (agonists) or prevent its activation by a naturally occurring agonist (antagonists). One of the best examples of this is the beta adrenoreceptor, for which the natural agonists are adrenaline or noradrenaline. Agonists such as salbutamol are used to stimulate the receptor, specifically the beta 2 subtype, and cause bronchodilation or vasodilation, and we use antagonists such as propranolol (nonspecific) or atenolol (relatively beta 1 specific) to treat angina or hypertension. Many other drugs act at receptors: histamine H1 and H2 antagonists (e.g. terfenadine or cimetidine), opiates (e.g. diamorphine), benzodiazepines (e.g. diazepam), serotonin antagonists (e.g. ondansetron). Clearly, using two drugs with opposing actions at the same receptor would be nonsense.

Receptors can change in both number and sensitivity. Both increase if a patient is treated with an antagonist: this is called upregulation. For example, betablockers cause upregulation of the beta adrenoceptor, which may be why patients get a rebound overactivity when betablockers are withdrawn, possibly leading to an anginal attack. Conversely, prolonged exposure to an agonist leads to downregulation of the receptor, e.g. in heart failure, patients are chronically exposed to high levels of adrenaline and lose their sensitivity to it.

Other drugs act by inhibiting enzymes: for instance omeprazole which prevents hydrogen ion production in the parietal cells of the stomach, allopurinol which inhibits xanthine oxidase and blocks the formation of the insoluble uric acid, and monoamine oxidase inhibitors which are used to treat depression. Some drugs replace a missing natural substance, such as L-dopa. Others act on excitable cell membranes to influence impulse conduction, for instance antiarrhythmics or anticonvulsants.

Potency and efficacy

'Potency' refers to the dose of a drug needed to achieve a desired effect. If drug A is more potent than drug B, all this means is that the dose is lower for a given effect, e.g. bumetamide is more potent than frusemide and equivalent doses are 1 mg and 40 mg respectively. Potency is, therefore, of little clinical relevance. What is more important is the efficacy of a drug, i.e. the maximum effect which the drug is capable of achieving. Drug A (bumeta-mide) and drug B have equal efficacy, which is greater than that of drug C; but drug C is more potent than drug B (i.e. 2.5 mg of bendrofluazide gives a greater diuresis than 2.5 mg of frusemide, but frusemide has greater efficacy than bendrofluazide). This concept is often not understood by doctors, who may be misled, for instance, into thinking that 2.5 mg of lorazepam is a very low dose, and happily prescribe it two or three times per day. Those doctors would be horrified to be told that they were prescribing the equivalent of 25 mg of diazepam each time, as lorazepam is eight to ten times more potent than diazepam.

What the body does to drugs

This is sometimes called pharmacokinetics, and refers to the absorption, distribution, metabolism and excretion of drugs, i.e. how drugs get into the body, what happens once they are in, and how the body gets rid of them.

Absorption

Most drugs in general practice are given orally. Drugs may also be given by injection (parenterally), or topically, e.g. skin creams. Sometimes a drug is applied topically not just for a local effect but for a systemic effect, e.g. HRT patches. Drugs taken orally enter the stomach; some drugs are absorbed directly in the stomach such as alcohol and perhaps, to some extent, acidic drugs such as aspirin. Most pass through the stomach and are for the most part absorbed in the small intestine. The small intestine has such a huge surface area that only drastic reductions in the length of the small bowel or in its surface area (for instance in severe coeliac disease) will have any effect on absorption.

Most drugs are absorbed by passive diffusion, in that they pass through the lipid membrane of the mucosal cell walls passively. A small number use existing active absorption mechanisms, e.g. L-dopa. Most drugs are not completely absorbed – some are lost in the large bowel where they may have side effects, e.g. ampicillin causing diarrhoea. Once absorbed, the drug enters the portal venous system which carries it to the liver and then to the systemic circulation. Many drugs undergo some metabolism before entering the systemic circulation, either in the wall of the bowel or the liver. This is called first-pass metabolism, and its extent may vary from person to person. The term bioavailability describes the amount of the drug administered that reaches the systemic circulation (after absorption and first-pass metabolism) and is usually expressed as a percentage.

Distribution

Once a drug reaches the systemic circulation it is distributed around the body. Some drugs have an affinity for tissues while others stay in blood, depending on their physicochemical properties. Pharmacologists use the term 'apparent volume of distribution' to describe the theoretical volume of fluid needed to dissolve the drug to achieve the concentration measured in plasma. Drugs with a large volume of distribution (e.g. tricyclics, 70–80 l) are bound to tissues. This concept is useful in calculating clearances of drugs and what the drug binds to, but is not of any great value to prescribers.

Metabolism

Many lipid soluble drugs are metabolized in the body. Metabolism usually detoxifies or inactivates drugs, but some drugs are activated by metabolism, e.g. enalapril has to be metabolized to enalaprilat before it becomes active. Metabolism may occur in the liver or elsewhere, such as the lung or the kidney. The enzymes responsible for metabolism are very nonspecific, and deal with a wide range of endogenous products and exogenous toxins as well as drugs. The rates of metabolism depend on a range of factors, including the nutritional state, the genetically-determined complement of enzymes, any disease affecting the liver (although the liver has such a huge reserve of metabolizing capacity that only in severe liver disease is drug metabolism affected), or other vital organs. A further factor is the state of induction or inhibition of liver enzymes. Many drugs, such as carbamazepine, phenytoin, or rifampicin, and other substances such as alcohol or tobacco smoke, can induce or encourage the production of additional enzymes. This in turn enhances the liver's ability to metabolize some other drug, creating a risk of drug interactions, with decreased activity of the second drug. It takes time to produce the new protein enzymes and it can be approximately two weeks before any clinical consequence is seen.

Conversely, some other drugs act as enzyme inhibitors, and prevent the metabolism of other drugs. Examples of liver enzyme inhibitors include erythromycin, ciprofloxacin, and cimetidine. Inhibition occurs almost immediately, and again may cause serious drug interactions.

There are genetic differences in drug metabolizing enzymes. This is best described for drug acetylation. For instance in the metabolism of isoniazid, slow metabolizers (e.g. most Scandinavians and Egyptians) are at risk of peripheral neuropathy, while fast metabolizers (e.g. most Eskimo) are at risk of a poor therapeutic response and hepatitis. The British population is about half and half. Many other examples exist and new examples are being defined constantly.

Elimination

This refers to how the body stops the action of a drug, either by metabolizing it or by excreting it. The kidney is responsible for elimination of most water soluble drugs or metabolites. Renal elimination may be passive – when the drug is just excreted during glomerular filtration, e.g. gentamicin. Passive back diffusion may also occur, depending in part on whether the drug exists in an ionized state or as a neutral compound. We exploit this in treating overdose of aspirin; elimination of aspirin is enhanced by alkalinizing the urine, increasing the dissociation of aspirin and reducing its diffusion back into the systemic circulation. Excretion may be active – when the drug is actively secreted into the renal tubule, e.g. weak acids such as penicillin (sometimes we deliberately block this excretion with probenecid to give a longer effect). The elimination of some drugs by the kidney may be slowed by renal disease, and dose reduction may be necessary.

Half-life

Most drugs are cleared from the body exponentially, i.e. the more drug that is present, the more is cleared, and the elimination of a drug is described by its half-life, or the time taken for the plasma concentration to fall by half. This may give some idea of the duration of action of a drug, but plasma drug concentrations do not often reflect concentration at the receptor or receptor occupancy, and this is often impossible to measure. For instance, the half-life of atenolol is eight to nine hours. Nevertheless, atenolol usually gives adequate betablockade after a single dose for 18–24 hours. Also, some drugs have active metabolites which may be important in determining the duration of action of a drug. e.g. diazepam has a half-life of 20–50 hours but its active metabolite desmethydiazepam has a half-life of up to eight days.

Elimination of drug from the body is 97% complete after five half-lives. Conversely, it takes five half-lives for plasma concentrations of a drug to reach steady state in chronic administration.

Therapeutic window and therapeutic drug monitoring

The range of plasma concentrations within which we have a desired therapeutic response without undue toxicity is called the therapeutic window. For most drugs, this window is wide and so we do not monitor the drug concentration. For some drugs, the window is narrow, i.e. the plasma concentration at which we achieve the therapeutic response is very close to that at which the drug is toxic. For such drugs, we carefully monitor dose and measure response to dose either in its effects (e.g. prothrombin time and warfarin) or plasma concentration (e.g. digoxin, theophylline, lithium, some anticonvulsants, cyclosporin). A therapeutic range of plasma concentration is defined within which we should achieve our effect without toxicity, but in reality, such a range may not apply to the individual patient: some will have toxicity within the therapeutic range, and others will not have the desired effect until the plasma concentration is above the therapeutic range. The plasma concentration of such drugs is a guide to be interpreted cautiously along with patient response and evidence of toxicity.

Variation in drug response

Why don't all patients respond to the same dose of drug? We have seen several reasons, including variations in how the body handles the drug, and in the sensitivity of the body to drugs. Other factors include whether the patient actually takes the drug, the placebo response, and the physiological state of the patient.

Compliance

Most doctors assume that patients take drugs as prescribed, though they can never manage to complete a five-day course of antibiotics themselves. The reality is that only about 50–75% of long-term therapy is taken. This is true, even in serious illnesses such as epilepsy or TB, where failure to take a drug may lead to disease breakthrough. Causes for noncompliance include adverse effects, inconvenience, excessively complex therapeutic regimens and failure of the doctor to convince the patient that the benefits of long-term therapy exceed the inconvenience. Patients may not admit to noncompliance lest they offend the doctor. Not all noncompliance is deviant behaviour – some of it may be self-preservation by the patient from the excessive enthusiasms of their doctor.

Doctors need to be aware of the problem and to consider it a cause of therapeutic failure, and should work to minimize the risks. Simple drug regimens are important. Compliance is better with drugs taken once or twice a day than with those taken three or more times a day. Single drug therapy is likely to be better than more complex regimes. Informing the patient of the nature and aims of therapy (repeatedly, and in writing) is also important.

Influences of disease and age on response to drug therapy

Some disease states affect response to drugs. These changes can occur as a result of a change in plasma levels of the drugs (pharmacokinetic), or in the response to a given drug concentration (pharmacodynamic). Examples of pharmacokinetic effects include increased drug concentrations of, for instance, digoxin, and toxicity in patients with renal disease on standard doses. Examples of pharmacodynamic effects include the sensitivity of patients with liver disease to opiates or benzodiazepines. Other examples include increased drug concentrations of lipid-soluble drugs in patients with congestive cardiac failure (due to decreased liver blood flow).

The old are generally more sensitive to drugs. Renal function declines with age and slower excretion of a drug may lead to higher plasma concentrations. Liver function, in contrast, is usually well preserved, although the elderly are more sensitive to warfarin. There are also pharmacodynamic changes, which are not well understood. The elderly are more sensitive to benzodiazepines and to antihypertensives. They are generally prone to adverse effects (see Chapter 2), in part because they are (not always wisely) prescribed more drugs.

Formulation

Drugs can be administered in many forms. In general practice they are most commonly given orally, in the form of tablets or capsules. Only a small proportion of the tablet/capsule actually contains an active drug – the remainder is made up of excipients, such as inert material like lactose, and colouring and binding agents. Excipients, which often are not identified on package labelling, can sometimes give rise to adverse effects.

Some patients find tablets difficult to swallow. They should be advised to take them while sitting up and with a drink of water. Capsules are generally easier to take. Soluble preparations also avoid this problem.

Some tablets contain the active drug in a modified release form designed to slow down and prolong its release. This may have advantages: the adverse effects may, in part, have been due to high peak concentration, and so this is avoided; the longer duration of action may also prolong the dosing interval and reduce the number of tablets a patient needs to take, and this may in turn improve compliance. In general, the latter advantage is overplayed by the manufacturers.

Other formulations are designed to be taken sublingually, bypassing the first pass metabolism since the blood supply to the mucosa under the tongue goes to the systemic circulation rather than into the portal circulation (e.g. glyceryl trinitrate). Other ways to administer drugs that bypass first pass metabolism are transcutaneously, or rectally by suppository.

Conclusion

An understanding of the basics of clinical pharmacology goes a long way towards understanding what we are actually doing when we prescribe a drug. While one can survive without this knowledge, one then tends to prescribe by rote, without really considering the patient or the drug: this is surely the essence of irrational prescribing.

Further reading

Feely J and Brodie M. (1991) Drug handling and response. *New Drugs* (2nd edn), ed. J. Feely, BMJ, London.
Walley T and Scott AK. (1995) Prescribing in the elderly. *Postgraduate Medical Journal*; 71: 466–71.

2　Adverse drug reactions and drug interactions

Tom Walley

Adverse drug reactions

Adverse drug reactions (ADRs) can be defined as any unintended harmful effect of a drug. They have replaced diseases such as syphilis or tuberculosis as the great mimics. The rate of adverse drug reactions in patients taking drugs is higher than many doctors suspect. It is estimated that ADRs occur in 10–20% of all patients prescribed drugs and are the cause of up to 10% of all GP consultations, 4% of all hospital admissions and 6–10% of admissions to geriatric wards, and about one in 1000 deaths. Importantly, up to half of drug reactions leading to hospital admissions are due to inappropriate drug therapy, i.e. the use of contraindicated or interacting drugs, or unnecessary drugs. Patients may not report these ADRs to their doctors, either because they accept them as part of their disease or treatment, or because they do not wish to offend the doctor. Both doctors and patients must accept that *all* drugs carry risks of adverse reactions. Sir Derrick Dunlop who founded the Committee on Safety of Medicines commented that any drug that does not cause adverse effects is probably totally ineffective. Patients sometimes do not understand these risks, but inexcusably, neither, it seems, do some doctors.

All prescribing is therefore a matter of weighing the risks and benefits of the use of a drug: when the benefits outweigh the risks, we prescribe, and when the risks outweigh the benefits, we do not. Sometimes this is a difficult judgement. It is important to explain the difficult decision to the patient, and seek their understanding and agreement. As a routine, when prescribing, doctors should mention the common and the major adverse effects to their patients. Many doctors may feel that they should not worry their patients in this way (and in some cases this is a reasonable approach), but in general, how else can a patient be said to have given informed consent for the treatment? For their own protection, doctors should record such conversations in the patients' case notes.

Classification

Adverse drug reactions can be classified into four broad types:

Type A: the augmented or attenuated effect, where the ADR is due to an excessive or inadequate pharmacological effect of the drug. These may be due to pharmacokinetic or pharmacodynamic problems. In either case, the ADR is predictable from the known effects of the drug and is dose related, e.g. hypotension in patients taking antihypertensives, or excessive sedation in a patient taking carbamazepine. Such effects are very common, but are often not severe. Type A ADRs can be managed or avoided often by simple modification of the dose.

Type B: the bizarre effect, which is not predictable from the known effects of the drug and often has an immunological basis. There is usually no clear relationship to the dose of drug. Such ADRs are relatively rare, but are disproportionately important because the ADR is often very serious, e.g. anaphylaxis with penicillin, or agranulocytosis with carbimazole. Complete withdrawal of the drug is necessary for treatment, as well as avoiding future exposure to it.

Type C: the effects of chronic administration of a drug, usually due to adaptation to the drug, or change in the sensitivity of receptors, e.g. rebound angina on withdrawal of betablockers because of upregulation of beta adrenoceptors (see Chapter 1), or the on/off phenomenon with L-dopa.

Type D: delayed effects, such as carcinogenesis or effects on reproduction, e.g. stilboestrol, which caused adenocarcinoma of the vagina in the daughters of women who had taken it while pregnant.

How do we learn about adverse drug reactions?

Our ability to identify an ADR in an individual patient may depend on whether we are aware of its possibility. So how do we identify new adverse reactions, not previously described, or estimate the risks of adverse reactions?

Pre-marketing drug testing

During drug development, a new drug will be given to an average of about 1500 healthy people (this number continues to rise as drug testing becomes more rigorous). This early testing will show up many common ADRs, especially ADRs of type A. However, type B reactions may be rare, perhaps with an incidence of only one in 10 000 or less, and so are unlikely to be seen in early drug trials. These ADRs may become apparent only after the drug is marketed and widely prescribed, and the number of patients treated with it rises. Likewise the late type C and D effects are only likely to be seen after the drug has been available for some years. It may be difficult to connect an adverse event with the drug, especially if the ADR resembles other disease, e.g. liver damage on perhexilene, an antianginal drug now withdrawn, caused histological changes identical to those due to alcoholism and was not recognized as an ADR for some years.

After marketing

The yellow card

It is important, therefore, when new drugs are prescribed, that doctors observe closely for any possible adverse effect and report it to the Committee on Safety of Medicines (CSM). This is the statutory body responsible for assessing the safety of drugs before they are licensed and for collecting reports of adverse reactions afterwards. Reports to the CSM can be made on special yellow cards, which are widely available in the BNF, in FP10 pads and in the compendium of drug data sheets. The CSM asks for reports of all serious adverse reactions or suspected adverse reactions to any drug, and for special reporting of all suspected adverse reactions to newly-introduced drugs. These drugs are marked in the BNF or in promotional literature with a black triangle (▼). The importance of this cannot be overstressed. New drugs are regularly withdrawn because doctors suspected previously undescribed adverse reactions to them and reported them. Examples in the recent past include the antibiotic temofloxacin which caused unexpected liver disturbances, and terodiline, used to treat urinary incontinence in the elderly, which caused cardiac arrhythmias. Other serious reactions that this system was vital in identifying include venous thromboembolic disease by oral contraceptives. It has had its failures too – it was slow to identify the risk of dependency to benzodiazepines. This illustrates the weakness of such a system: unless a doctor suspects a problem, he cannot report it. Rates of reporting of adverse reactions can be influenced by publicity surrounding it. For example, the CSM acted to withdraw terodiline after receiving six reports of cardiac arrhythmias: after its withdrawal, over thirty further reports were received as doctors suddenly realized that they too had seen a case.

Although the CSM receives about 20 000 reports per year, only a tiny fraction of adverse reactions is ever reported. Doctors usually excuse themselves for not reporting by saying they did not think of the possibility of an adverse reaction, or did not have a yellow card handy, or meant to do it later and forgot. The biggest reason is that doctors simply do not appreciate how important such reporting is.

Post-marketing surveillance

It is increasingly common for the licensing authority to include, as a condition of its licensing, a requirement that the company conducts a specific post-marketing safety surveillance study. The aims of these studies is to observe the effects of the use of the drug in everyday practice and detect adverse reactions. Such studies will often involve several thousand patients who are given the drug on its clinical merits in the usual way and then the outcome is observed. Given the numbers of patients involved, companies usually need to secure the cooperation of general practitioners, who may be paid a small fee for their help. In the past, such studies were used as a means of drug promotion, effectively paying doctors for entering patients into the trial and so encouraging the use of the drug. Of course such trials are unethical, and with better monitoring should be rare today; doctors must consider the ethics of any trial they are asked to participate in (see Chapter 15).

There is a range of other means of assessing the frequency of adverse drug reactions. The post-event monitoring (PEM) green card system identifies GPs who have prescribed the drug of interest, and asks them to report any adverse event which the patient subsequently suffered: although many such events have nothing to do with the drug, some may. This gets around the problem of doctors not realizing that they are seeing an adverse effect. GP computer systems contain a wealth of drug safety data derived from experience and are increasingly used for this by epidemiologists.

Patients particularly at risk of ADRs

Some patients are particularly at risk from adverse reactions and merit special caution in prescribing. They include:

- the elderly – who have little physiological reserve so that they are less likely to tolerate, for instance, minor falls in blood pressure. They also have altered pharmacokinetics and pharmacodynamics, as explained in the previous chapter

- the very young

- patients with renal disease

- patients with liver disease

- genetically-predisposed patients, e.g. patients with glucose 6-phosphate dehydrogenase deficiency, who may get haemolysis when treated with many drugs such as sulphonamides, or antimalarials such as primaquine, or patients with acute intermittent porphyria who may get exacerbations if given many drugs (e.g. oestrogens) that are metabolized by the liver and interfere with haem breakdown.

Every doctor recognizes patients who seem to get adverse effects on every drug which they are prescribed. While this is possible, one has to suspect that either the doctor is prescribing in a bizarre way (such as always prescribing at the top of the dose range) or that the patient enjoys being a puzzle to medical science and defying all attempts to help him or her.

Drug interactions

We usually think of drug interactions as harmful, but they may, of course, be beneficial. Examples of beneficial interactions include that between L-dopa and benserazide which prevents the conversion of L-dopa to dopamine outside the CNS and so minimizes its adverse effects, or the ability of probenecid to block the excretion of penicillin. Not all of the many interactions described are of clinical importance, and like adverse drug reactions, clinically significant interactions may not occur in every patient prescribed potentially interacting drugs.

Many lists or charts of possible drug interactions are available. Rather than attempting to learn lists off by heart, it is better for the most part to consider:

- which patients are at risk

- which drugs are most likely to be involved

- what the possible mechanisms are.

GPs and pharmacists are now greatly helped by the use of computers, for prescribing in general practice, and for dispensing in community pharmacies. Simple interaction programmes should avoid most of the potentially harmful interactions. Nevertheless, constant vigilance is required to avoid interactions and to spot them when they do occur. Some common or dangerous interactions are mentioned below, but the list is not complete: check carefully before prescribing if there is any doubt.

Patients who are at risk of interactions

1   The elderly – largely because of polypharmacy: the average patient over

the age of 65 receives 16 prescriptions per year, and in surveys, the number of concurrent drugs in those prescribed regular therapy ranged from 2.7 to 4.8 in the 65–74 year old patients, and from 3.2 to 6.7 in those aged 75–84. Other factors include multiple morbidity, poor homeostatic mechanisms and the pharmacokinetic and dynamic changes already discussed.

2   Severely ill patients – again, they may have little reserve and be prescribed many drugs, but also because a drug interaction may be difficult to distinguish from the natural history of the disease, e.g. heart failure treated with diuretics may be exacerbated by NSAIDs which cause fluid retention.

3   Patients who depend on prophylactic therapy or disease suppression – e.g. epileptics, patients on immunosuppressants, or oral contraceptives. Interactions may lead to disease breakthrough.

4   Patients with liver or renal disease.

5   Patients with more than one doctor – where confusion may arise over what drugs the patient is taking (confusion between doctors and also between doctors and patient – this is especially important for instance between hospital doctors and general practitioners).

6   Patients who take nonprescribed drugs – e.g. those bought 'over the counter' such as theophylline, cimetidine, pseudoephedrine in decongestants and, of course, ethanol – and who often do not tell their doctor about these drugs because they do not consider them to be real drugs or because they do not want to admit they are taking them.

Risk drugs

Some drugs are particularly likely to be involved in serious interactions.

- Drugs with a narrow therapeutic index, e.g. warfarin, digoxin, cytotoxics, lithium, aminoglycosides, theophylline.

- Drugs with a steep dose–response curve, where a minor change in plasma concentration may make a major change in effect, e.g. oral hypoglycaemics, warfarin.

- Drugs with a major effect on a vital process such as clotting (warfarin).

- Drugs where a loss of effect may lead to disease breakthrough, e.g. antiepileptics.

- Drugs that may induce or inhibit enzymes responsible for metabolizing drugs, and so may increase or decrease metabolism of other drugs (see below for examples of such drugs).

- Drugs which depend on these enzymes for their metabolism (e.g. theophylline, warfarin, phenytoin, oral contraceptives, cyclosporin and many others).

Mechanisms

Drug interactions may be pharmacokinetic or pharmacodynamic.

Pharmacokinetic

Where the interaction causes a change in the plasma concentration of one or other drug leading to a greater or lesser effect.

1   Absorption: drugs such as cholestyramine may bind to other drugs (e.g. digoxin, thiazides) in the gastrointestinal tract and prevent their absorption.

    Some drugs undergo enterohepatic circulation, i.e. they are excreted in a conjugated form in bile. The conjugation is broken down by bacteria in the bowel and the free drug is reabsorbed, enhancing drug effect, e.g. oral contraceptive oestrogens. If this is prevented, e.g. by amoxycillin altering gut flora, the drug may lose its effect.

2   Metabolism: enzyme inducers (e.g. phenytoin, carbamazepine, rifampicin) will decrease the effects of many drugs; since enzyme induction requires synthesis of new protein, it may take two to three weeks to reach its maximum effect. Enzyme inhibitors on the other hand (erythromycin, ciprofloxacin, isoniazid, cimetidine, sodium valproate, metronidazole, allopurinol, dextropropoxyphene, sulphonamides and many others) are effective very rapidly. Problems may arise therefore when a patient stable on a drug is prescribed either an enzyme inducer or inhibitor. Problems may also arise if a patient is stabilized on a drug while receiving an enzyme inducer or inhibitor which is then withdrawn.

3   Distribution: only free drug is pharmacologically active, but many drugs are heavily protein bound, e.g. warfarin to albumin. If another drug with a high affinity for protein is prescribed, the result may be a displacement of warfarin from the protein-binding sites, increasing the free drug and its effects. This is usually a transient effect since the body clears free

drug, and the increased free drug is cleared more rapidly until a steady state is restored.

4   Excretion: thiazides and NSAIDs interfere with the excretion of lithium. This type of interaction can also be beneficial; e.g. reducing the clearance of penicillin by probenecid.

Pharmacodynamic

These interactions are predictable from the known effects of the drug, e.g. two antihypertensives may be used to lower the blood pressure more than either can alone. Alternatively, the actions of diuretics are opposed by NSAIDs which may cause fluid retention, or the effects of oral hypoglycaemics may be opposed by thiazides. Other pharmacodynamic interactions can arise from the effect of drugs in electrolyte or fluid balance, e.g. diuretic induced hypokalaemia enhances digoxin toxicity. Sometimes doctors mistakenly simultaneously prescribe drugs with opposite actions at a receptor e.g. a beta agonist like salbutamol with a beta antagonist like atenolol.

Conclusion

Adverse drug reactions are common and are under-recognized by doctors. Adverse reactions may be an important factor in poor compliance. Fortunately most adverse reactions are fairly mild, but some may cause serious morbidity or even death. New drugs may have serious adverse effects which are not yet recognized, and should be prescribed with caution. Doctors should report all adverse effects to new drugs and all serious adverse effects, even if well recognized, using yellow cards. Drug interactions are also important and must be considered, especially where high-risk patients are on high-risk drugs.

Further reading

Bateman D and Chaplin S. (1991) Adverse reactions to drugs. *New drugs* (2nd edn), ed. Feely J, *BMJ*, London.
Brodie M and Feely J. (1991) Adverse drug interactions. *New drugs* (2nd edn), ed. Feely J, *BMJ*, London.

Davies D M (ed). (1991) *Textbook of adverse drug reactions* (4th edn), Oxford University Press, Oxford.
Griffin J P, D'Arcy P F, Speirs C J. (1988) *A manual of adverse drug interactions* (3rd edn), Wright, London.

3   Taking responsibility

Peter R Fellows

Prescriber beware! A signature on a prescription signifies much more than just an order to supply a particular drug, dressing or appliance. It implies acceptance of responsibility for that action and an understanding of what is being prescribed, what beneficial effects may be expected, and what other effects, including side effects, allergic potential, and interactions may occur.

Under his or her terms of service, a general practitioner is expected to demonstrate only the degree of knowledge that general practitioners as a class would be expected to have. Many GPs have specialized skills and knowledge, related to their special interests and their training. If they choose to prescribe on the basis of that special knowledge, then they are individually accountable.

Who can prescribe?

Consultants and GPs may prescribe for private or NHS patients. Dentists and approved nurses may prescribe, but have restricted prescribing lists. A GP may receive prescribing advice from a consultant, a nurse, a Macmillan nurse, an optician, or a physiotherapist, for example, but it is important to differentiate between advice given to the GP to assist his personal management and a request to prescribe on behalf of someone else who wishes to retain the clinical responsibility. Once a GP prescribes he is accepting the clinical and legal responsibility for his action.

A GP may be pressurized to supply signed blank prescriptions, or completed prescriptions for an unnamed patient. For example a midwife may plead that she does not like to bother the doctor every time for prescriptions for iron or antacids. This should be resisted. Doctors have been known to leave blank signed prescriptions at a local pharmacy. A signature on a blank prescription could land the doctor before the GMC. Beware! In a case of urgency the GP's terms of service entitle him to request a chemist to dispense a drug or appliance before a prescription is issued, provided it is not a controlled drug, and provided he undertakes to furnish the chemist with a prescription within 72 hours.

Whether to prescribe or not to prescribe

The responsible prescriber first has to decide whether to prescribe at all. It is more appropriate to stop the NSAID that has caused oedema, than to prescribe a diuretic. It is sometimes easy, under the pressure of a busy surgery, to write a prescription for a drug when the patient is already taking a very similar one. The GP should always check what the patient is already taking. There is a trend to make more 'prescription only medicines' available over the counter. The doctor will be culpable if his patient has a haematemesis following a prescription for an NSAID, when he did not realize that the patient was already taking Nurofen!

A GP is required to issue an NHS prescription (FP10) for any drugs or appliances that are needed for the treatment of his NHS patients. The exception to this is where a drug has been 'blacklisted' and is included in schedule 10 of the regulations (see Chapter 10). Then a doctor may not issue an FP10 prescription, but may issue a private prescription. Schedule 11 is similar but permits FP10 prescription of the included drugs for treatment of specified conditions only. The doctor must endorse the FP10 with the reference 'SLS'. Problems may result because these restrictions do not apply to hospital doctors. Recently, carbocisteine was prescribed for an elderly hemiplegic who lives alone, is confined to a wheelchair, and who had been discharged from hospital after a laryngectomy. The drug was started by the consultant. The drug is on schedule 11, permitted for tracheostomy patients, but it had been forgotten that it is allowed only for patients up to the age of 18. The patient must now obtain the drug from the District General Hospital (DGH) 22 miles away, or the GP will be liable for the cost. Such pitfalls wait to trap the prescriber. Beware!

The Department of Health has indicated that a GP may prescribe privately if a prescription only medicine would cost less than the prescription charge. The doctor cannot be sure what the chemist might charge for dispensing the prescription, and the patient may end up paying more than the prescription charge would have been on an FP10. He may then make a complaint against the doctor. Unless the Government changes the regulations, an FP10 should be issued.

The GP cannot treat a patient on his list privately. Neither may he issue an FP10 to a patient in the course of private treatment. A consultant who sees a patient privately may advise on appropriate drugs for further management by the GP. The GP may then issue an FP10. Sometimes, however, the consultant is continuing private treatment that he is supervising, and in such circumstances the drugs should be supplied by the consultant on private prescription. The patient, issued with a private prescription, may approach the GP and ask for an FP10 to be substituted. In these circumstances the GP is entitled to refuse.

Writing the prescription

Badly written prescriptions are a common factor in complaints. Beware! A prescription should be legible. The patient must be clearly identified. Surname, initial, one full forename, and address are necessary. The age of the patient must be written for a child of under twelve. Recently the Government has suggested that we should put the age of the patient on every prescription, as a means of policing prescription charge fraud where patients give false information about their age. That would involve yet another task, and could lead to complaint if a mistake is made and the patient is wrongly charged, or not charged, by the pharmacist.

The item ordered on the prescription, and the form in which it is to be dispensed, must be clearly specified, along with the total quantity. It is best to avoid abbreviations where possible, and to write the strength in grams (g), milligrams (mg), or micrograms. Micrograms should be written out in full to avoid confusion. It is best not to use decimal points, e.g. 0.25 g is better written as 250 mg. Ideally there should be specific directions for the use of the item prescribed, and sometimes specific warnings. The prescription should be dated and it must be signed in ink. Carbon copies, excluding the signature, are acceptable except in the case of controlled drugs. Rubber stamps and computer generated signatures are not acceptable. The form in which the medication should be dispensed requires common sense. Recently a doctor was fined for prescribing enteric-coated prednisolone tablets for a two year old child. His assertion that he meant the tablets to be crushed was not accepted.

Commissioning Authority medical advisers are policing over-prescribing. There are some blatant cases, but there is no precise definition of what constitutes over-prescribing. Some doctors are prescribing 12 months supply of the contraceptive pill at one time. This could be challenged on the grounds of possible waste. A doctor was recently criticized by a service committee for prescribing three months supply of a drug within weeks of issuing a similar prescription, having inadvertently pressed an additional print button on his computer. Beware!

Pharmacists would prefer a maximum prescription of 28 days supply (one problem with prepacked 'monitored dosage' schemes). There is no need for such a limited supply for many chronic stable conditions, and there are serious implications both for the doctor's workload and the patient's pocket.

Commissioning Authority managers are setting targets for generic prescribing. Coercion is occurring in some places with threats to funding for staff reimbursement and premises. There are complex issues involved in generic prescribing, and it is not necessarily always a good thing, or cheaper in the long run for the Government. There is no requirement for a GP to prescribe generically except for some substances affected by the 'blacklist'.

A GP was recently fined £1000 by a service committee. He had been asked by telephone during a busy surgery if he would prescribe penicillin for a recurrent 'tonsillitis'. He was put under some pressure by the patient who had an important engagement. It is not normally this doctor's policy to prescribe antibiotics for sore throats, but he agreed. He used his computer to prescribe, and typed in 'PEN', which brought up a picking list. He selected the number for penicillin 'V' and signed the prescription. He did not notice that he had entered the wrong number and that the computer had printed 'penicillamine'. Fortunately the patient came to no harm. The case illustrates potential pitfalls with computer generated prescriptions, as well as the confusion that can arise through very similar generic names.

Schedule 10, the 'blacklist', permits the FP10 prescription of some substances, such as diazepam, only when prescribed generically. If the doctor is uncertain he is advised to check in the BNF or MIMS where a 'g' is listed alongside the affected drug, or a cross if it is blacklisted in all forms. Such checks are irritating and time consuming, but may prevent the doctor being charged for the drug. Other substances, known as 'borderline substances', are regarded as drugs only in the treatment of certain conditions. Prescription for these items will not usually be challenged if the prescription is endorsed 'ACBS', which indicates the doctor's awareness that he is prescribing for an approved condition. Many nutritional products and cosmetics are borderline substances.

The GP is required by his terms of service to keep adequate records of his patient's illness and treatment.

Computer generated prescriptions

The information obtained from a computer is only as good as the information put in. Beware! Computers have many advantages. They produce legible prescriptions and provide lists of authorized repeat prescriptions, possible interactions and dates of previous prescriptions. Messages, such as a need to make an appointment, can be printed on the fly sheet. Repeat prescribing can be much better supervised. Substitution of generic names, which might otherwise be difficult to remember, is easy. Audit and research are facilitated. Patients with conditions such as epilepsy or hypothyroidism can be traced by a computer search based on drugs prescribed.

Confusion can occur if the repeat prescription list is not kept up to date. It is not unusual to find several different NSAIDs or contraceptive pills on one patient's authorized list. Hurried signature of batches of computer generated repeat prescriptions can be hazardous for the unwary doctor. All prescriptions should be properly checked. The doctor is responsible if an error occurs.

Security

It is the responsibility of the doctor to ensure that prescription pads are securely stored, and that pads are not left lying around on reception counters or consulting room desks. They are valuable to a thief. If signed prescriptions are left for collection, possibly at a branch surgery, they should be secure from theft.

Access to computer information also needs consideration. It is wise to change security log-in codes at intervals.

Advice to the patient

Advice to a patient to use a particular community pharmacist is unethical. Care must be taken over any arrangements for collection and delivery services, since the patient has the right to choose which pharmacist to use.

The prescriber must give appropriate advice to the patient about the drugs prescribed. He should explain what the drug is intended to do, check on possible allergy, and point out possible adverse effects. A severe reaction to amoxycillin when hypersensitivity to penicillin is recorded on the notes would be indefensible. He must be aware of possible interactions and warn the patient appropriately. Problems occur with alcohol, especially increased sedation. The contraceptive pill may be affected by antibiotics and anticonvulsants, leading to unwanted pregnancy. The doctor is vulnerable to complaint and it is a good habit to record that advice has been given. Routinely write in the margin, for example, 'WRD' (warned re drink, drowsiness, driving), or 'WROCP' (warned re oral contraceptive pill). Pregnancy, or the possibility of it, and lactation, must also be considered before prescribing.

Patients are often surprisingly well informed, particularly if things go wrong. Medicines are often supplied with a manufacturer's information sheet, and this will be the norm with 'original pack' prescribing. Pharmacists often supply their own information leaflets, and their computers print standard warnings, which may cause confusion, such as advice not to take antacids if taking an NSAID.

Data sheet information can change, and the doctor is responsible for keeping himself up to date. A few years ago data sheets for co-trimoxazole were suddenly changed to list 'age over 70' as a contraindication, resulting in at least one doctor suffering a formal hearing because of an adverse reaction. The data sheet was soon changed back to remove the contraindication, and now simply requires 'caution in the elderly'.

The hospital–GP interface

The drugs that a patient takes into hospital are his personal property and should be returned to him with appropriate advice. There have been problems when a large supply of a drug has been taken from a patient on admission, and only a few days' supply of the same drug has been returned to him on discharge.

Hospitals are not restricted to the limitations of the FP10, the 'drug tariff', or 'blacklist'. Most now have formularies which may not include the brands of drug which a patient is admitted on. Many use generics extensively. Frequent problems occur with specialized dressings that are not available to the GP. Pharmaceutical companies may supply hospitals cheaply with a drug which will then be an unnecessarily expensive treatment for continued prescription by the GP.

One constant irritation has been the patient who is discharged with only a few days supply of medication, and no discharge letter. It is now expected by the Department of Health that at least seven days supply should be given, so that discharge information can reach the GP, and suitable arrangements for repeat prescribing can be made. This should be specified in Purchaser/ Provider contracts.

Clinical responsibility should determine responsibility for prescribing. There are many pressures on GPs' prescribing costs, and 'target' budgets could become 'fixed' budgets. In fundholding practices, hard-won savings from prescribing costs may be earmarked for other patient services. The Purchaser/Provider contracts should include the cost of prescribing within the overall package. In spite of this, cost shifting is still a recurring problem that may present the GP with moral dilemmas. With outpatient management it is not always easy to determine who has clinical responsibility. In some instances there may be genuinely shared care, and it is reasonable for the GP to prescribe. For complex cancer treatments and infertility programmes the extremely specialized nature of the treatment points clearly to the consultant. A GP who would not normally have the specialized knowledge to claim clinical responsibility may be asked to prescribe expensive treatments such as growth hormone, erythropoetin, GRH analogues or interferon. A recent ploy is for the consultant to issue a protocol. If a GP does not feel competent to supervise such specialized treatments, he is justified in insisting that the consultant prescribes. The difficulty comes if there is an inference that because of financial constraint the patient may not receive necessary treatment unless the GP agrees to prescribe. Such problems are now problems for Purchasers as much as for the GP, and help should be sought from the medical adviser at the Commissioning Authority.

Some expensive 'social' treatments, such as IVF, are excluded from NHS provision by some Commissioning Authorities. A patient who is not well off may have no alternative but to seek expensive private treatment if she wishes to have a family. The private clinic (some are subsidized by charities) may ask the GP to prescribe expensive courses of hormone drugs involved in the treatment. The GP has no clinical responsibility as such, and would be justified in refusing. Some Commissioning Authorities have refused to sanction such prescriptions in calculating prescribing budgets. Others have been more amenable. The GP faced with such a moral dilemma may agree to prescribe, but by doing so he accepts responsibility for his action.

Responsibility for cost

Responsible prescribing is not 'cheap' prescribing, but should be cost-effective prescribing. PACT information is readily available, not only to the GP, but also to medical advisers and managers. Budgets are designed to exert downward pressure on prescribing. The ability of fundholders to retain savings from prescribing economies, and the emergence of 'prescribing incentive' schemes leave GPs vulnerable to accusation. Recently the right to remove patients from lists has been threatened because of a misguided belief that patients are being removed on the grounds of expense.

Drugs for out-of-hours use

A GP is expected to provide drugs for out-of-hours use, and except in Scotland, receives a small capitation payment to pay for them. In Scotland a GP may prescribe drugs for his night bag.

Many GPs rely on samples provided by pharmaceutical companies for out-of-hours use. This can lead to expensive and inappropriate prescribing. Many GPs will use unwanted drugs which have been returned to the surgery. This practice is risky in the event of a problem, and the doctor should be aware of product liability law.

Dispensing doctors have the great advantage of constant access to a full range of drugs, but all GPs can dispense some items that they 'personally' administer. This includes injections used out of hours. Details are in paragraph 44 of the Statement of Fees and Allowances. Sutures, ring pessaries, contraceptive diaphragms, coils, some immunizations, diagnostic reagents, etc., are also available under the Paragraph 44 rule.

A pharmacist may be willing to dispense out of hours, and is paid extra for doing so if the prescription is marked urgent by the doctor. The Local Pharmaceutical Committee usually maintains a list of pharmacists who are willing to dispense out of hours.

Product liability law

Since March 1988 all doctors have been advised to keep a detailed record of all medicines dispensed in case of 'product liability' claims by the patient under the terms of the Consumer Protection Act. Such claims can be made up to ten years after the event. The patient does not have to prove negligence, merely that he has suffered some adverse effect due to, for instance, faulty manufacture of a medicine.

This particularly affects dispensing doctors, but applies to any doctor personally supplying drugs in an emergency or out of hours. Generic drugs may present special difficulty. If the manufacturer can be identified, responsibility passes to him. If not, the last link in the chain will be held responsible. That may well be the doctor. If a supplier of a generic drug has gone out of business it may not be possible to identify the manufacturer. For self-protection all GPs should keep records of suppliers of any drug or appliance that they give directly to the patient. Dispensing doctors should keep records of suppliers for all generics they dispense, and retain them for a period of 11 years. Care should be taken to ensure that any dispensed medicine is labelled correctly.

Bulk prescribing

A separate prescription form must be used for each patient. There is only one exception, and that is where a doctor is prescribing in bulk for a school or institution in which at least 20 persons reside, and where the doctor has at least ten of those persons on his list. He may prescribe for two or more of those persons on a single FP10. The doctor does not write the patients' names, but heads the prescription with the name of the institution (which must be registered with the Commissioning Authority), and the number of persons for whom he is prescribing. Bulk prescribing is restricted to drugs and appliances prescribable under the NHS, but excludes 'prescription-only medicines'. It may be useful, for example, in treating head lice at a boarding school.

Residential homes

A doctor may be asked to complete drug charts at a residential home. It is not part of his terms of service to do so, and an NHS GP is not permitted to charge a retainer for such services. The doctor may be prepared to cooperate, and that would be regarded as good practice. Doctors may be put under pressure to use 'monitored dosage systems'. Such systems can be very wasteful if medication changes. They should only ever be introduced with the full agreement of the doctor and pharmacist. The Royal Pharmaceutical Society of Great Britain produces a useful booklet *The Administration and Control of Medicines in Residential and Children's Homes*.

Foreign travel

The Department of Health clarified in 1993 that a GP is obliged to supply sufficient 'long term maintenance' medicines to cover a temporary trip abroad of up to three months duration. If a patient is intending to be abroad for more than three months, he ceases to be on the doctor's list as soon as he leaves the country. Then the doctor should only supply sufficient medicines for the patient to reach his destination and arrange an alternative supply. The Department of Health is amending regulations to bar antimalarial prophylactics on FP10. Some newer antimalarial drugs are prescription-only medicines and a private prescription must be given, but many antimalarials are available for purchase without prescription from a pharmacy. The pharmacist can advise patients on use of these.

'Just in case' medicines should not be prescribed on an FP10, but the doctor may write a private prescription.

Seeking advice

The Commissioning Authority medical adviser can be helpful, and the Commissioning Authority may well employ a pharmacy facilitator. The Local Medical Committee secretary has access to much information, and can obtain more detail if necessary from the General Medical Services Committee. This may be particularly useful where terms of service issues are concerned. The local DGH will probably have a drug information pharmacist. GPs should be aware of how to contact the local 'Poisons Centre'. Medical departments of pharmaceutical companies, listed in the back of *MIMS*, are useful for factual information on their products and on interactions. Do not forget your local consultants, or your local chemist. The chemist may well have an up-to-date copy of *Martindale*. Detailed levels of PACT analysis can be requested from the Prescription Pricing Authority (PPA).

MIMS, the *BNF*, and the *Data Sheet Compendium* should be on every doctor's desk. *Unless we take the responsibilities of prescribing seriously, restriction will be inevitable.*

4 Quality and measurement

Conrad M Harris

A great deal of effort is being made at the moment to find ways of measuring the quality of a practice's prescribing, but much of it is very unsatisfactory. This chapter deals with some of the issues involved and describes what real progress has been made.

Quality

There is no direct way of assessing the quality of a practice's prescribing. Each prescription is given to an individual patient: to judge its quality one would have to be sure that the diagnosis was correct and to know a great deal more about the patient. Even if this were possible, there could be dispute between the prescriber and the judge, since many traditional and generally accepted treatments fall a long way short of the ideal of evidence-based medicine.

The word 'quality' is used in different senses. Sometimes an absolute scale is implied: prescribing is 'good' or 'bad'. At other times it appeals to a concept of 'appropriateness for the purpose' – a relative judgement. A Rolls Royce, built to the highest standards, is not necessarily the best vehicle for transporting bags of manure – its qualities are inappropriate for the job, and its use is therefore open to criticism, even though the manure is transported effectively. In prescribing, arguments about 'absolute' quality tend to have a pharmacological basis, while those about 'relative' quality are likely to concern costs.

Because quality, in either sense, cannot be assessed directly, attention has been turned to ways of assessing it indirectly from prescribing data. This is logically possible only where everyone agrees that the use of a particular drug is 'bad' by absolute pharmacological standards. If such a drug is given frequently, the prescribing must be bad – but only in that particular respect; if it is not given at all, the prescribing is good – but again only in that respect. In neither case can any wider inferences about quality be drawn. We do not know yet whether prescribing that is bad in one such limited respect is particularly likely to be bad in others.

Quality indicators

Hundreds of different indicators based on prescribing data are being used across the country, with each Family Health Service Authority (FHSA) having its own, and it is usual to find them called quality indicators. Many of them are about cost, and stem from the relative definition of quality, but they tend to be mixed up with others that appeal to pharmacologically-based absolutes (sometimes very questionably), without any admission that two different standards are being invoked. An attempt to combine them under one heading is sometimes made by introducing the term 'rational' prescribing, in which both meanings of quality may have relevance. The problem is that rationality is such a powerful concept that its use obscures the fundamental weaknesses of any kind of indicator.

It has always been recognized by the thoughtful that indicators cannot be used for making judgements, and that they can do no more than point to areas that are worth discussing further with the practice involved. The practice may have a satisfactory or even a commendable reason for an indicator value that is high or low. Despite this, there is a temptation, not always resisted in a busy world, to turn the indicator value into a snap judgement. An explicit plan, stating how an indicator may be used, and what it will be used for, is required.

A development along these lines probably requires a change in the terminology to avoid confusion. A national group, working from Leeds, is proposing the more neutral 'prescribing indicator' or 'performance indicator'. It is finding only a small number of such indicators that stand up to scrutiny, and suggesting how they should be used. Each practice should be shown how it compares with the other practices in its FHSA, on each indicator, and invited to comment on its ranking. Any ranking about which it is unhappy may then become the subject of discussion. The best prescribing advisers will find nothing new in this approach, but its adoption as a universally observed procedure would represent progress.

It may be objected that this bypasses any notion of standards, or allows every practice to set its own, however idiosyncratically it may do so. While this is true, it has to be acknowledged that there are few areas in which standards can confidently be set. Even more importantly at the moment, the ways in which prescribing is measured are too imperfect for anyone to have much faith in the values ascribed to either the practice or the standard.

Measuring prescribing

At the moment, prescribing is usually measured in terms of three rates: the number of items per patient, the cost per item, and the cost per patient. These rates are applied both to prescribing overall and to prescribing in specific therapeutic groups. A practice's rates are compared with the average rates for all practices in its FHSA, and sometimes with national averages. None of these rates are satisfactory, and using FHSA averages as the standard for comparison is a very questionable procedure.

When the rates are used to compare FHSAs with each other, some patterns emerge. In the poorer, more industrial, areas, the items per patient rate tends to be relatively high and the cost per item relatively low. In more affluent areas, items per patient tends to be lower and cost per item higher. The cost per patient in both cases is determined more by the number of items than the cost of each item. When analyses of individual practices are made, however, not only is the variation much greater, but the patterns that were clear at FHSA level are lost. In searching for patterns that could be looked for at practice level, the Prescribing Research Unit soon became aware that part of the difficulty lay in the way prescribing was being measured.

Items

The number of items prescribed by a practice in a year depends to a considerable extent on the intended duration of the prescriptions. So little consistency in the number of tablets was found that a practice gave for particular drugs, in prescription duration in any FHSA, or in duration for particular drugs across practices, that we concluded that it was invalid to use number of items as a measurement unit. Intuitively, it seems wrong to regard a prescription for six tablets as equivalent to one for 600 tablets of the same drug.

Cost

This is also partly determined by the intended duration of the prescription, not just the costliness of the drug.

Patients

Different patients need different numbers of prescriptions: a practice population has to be standardized as far as possible to allow for this before fair comparisons can be made. Some allowance is given by the 'prescribing unit', which weights patients of 65 and over three times as heavily as younger patients, but the system is crude and no longer very accurate.

Rates based on these measures could not be reliable or valid, and this led to the work described on the following page.

Measuring a population

Prescribing is influenced by the age and sex structure of the population, so these factors have to be allowed for before a practice's prescribing can be understood or compared. The present 'prescribing unit' makes some allowance for age but is now not very accurate. A system was developed of ASTRO-PUs (age, sex and temporary resident originated prescribing units) that weights for nine age bands in both sexes, and for temporary residents, and this is now used in the setting of prescribing budgets. In time it will be used in PACT reports.

More recently similar cost-weightings for specific therapeutic groups have been established, because each group has a different age/sex distribution of use: cardiovascular and gastrointestinal drug costs are particularly high in older patients, endocrine drug costs are higher for women than for men, and antibiotics are given roughly equally to all age and sex groups, for example. These weightings are called STAR-PUs (specific therapeutic group age/sex related prescribing units), and they make possible much fairer comparators for a practice's prescribing than the kind of 'local averages' used at the moment.

Both ASTRO-PUs and STAR-PUs are based on the actual prescribing of large groups of practices; they do not incorporate any implication of quality or economy.

Measuring morbidity

The level of morbidity in a practice population must also influence prescribing, but there is no way of measuring it. Deprivation levels have therefore been used as a proxy for morbidity. The well-known Jarman index correlates poorly with prescribing costs, and in an attempt to do better the Low Income Scheme index was created. This is based on the percentage of prescribing costs for a population accounted for by items exempt from the prescription charge under one of the low income categories. Its advantages are that it can be updated frequently, it can be calculated for individual practices fairly easily, and it correlates with prescribing costs much better than the Jarman index does. It has, however, some deficiencies that make it suitable only for research purposes at the moment. No deprivation index is likely to account for very much of the variation between practices though, because the idiosyncratic habits of general practitioners tend to mask the effects of deprivation. The work continues.

Measuring prescribing volume

Defined daily doses (DDDs) provide a better way of measuring volume than the number of items prescribed, because they are independent of prescription duration. A DDD reflects the typical adult maintenance dosage of a drug per day, as set by the WHO. The value for ranitidine, for example, is 300 mg. This does not imply that all patients should receive 300 mg a day, but dividing the number of patients in the population by the number of 300 mg doses in a period of, say, a year gives a reasonable estimate of the rate at which ranitidine is given; this can be compared with the rates of other practices. The deliberately equivalent DDD for cimetidine is 800 mg, so it is meaningful to add the DDDs of ranitidine and cimetidine, plus those of similar drugs, to get a figure for ulcer healing preparations.

Though we have been working with the PPA to get DDDs on to its computers, we recognize several problems. Skin preparations and immunizations cannot have a DDD; paediatric dosages are ignored; and there are many technical problems to overcome. DDDs are international units, and, unfortunately, different countries sometimes use the same drug at different dosages. A few of the values set may therefore look odd over here. Similarly, some DDDs are set at the dosages used in hospital, and may be far higher than those prescribed by GPs.

A large study has been carried out to find out what dosages general practitioners here actually prescribe, and the aim is to produce a set of Standard Daily Doses (SDDs) that will be credible in this country as measures of volume.

Unmeasured factors

We are well aware that other factors may play a part in prescribing patterns, such as having patients in residential homes. These may have to be taken into account when a practice is negotiating its budget. The biggest unknown factor of all is probably doctors' idiosyncracies.

Conclusion

Progress is being made. It is becoming recognized that 'quality' is too difficult a concept to pursue very far, and that it is better to look for acceptable performance indicators that should be used educationally rather than punitively. The standardized measures being developed already reveal that an apparently high cost practice may in fact be more economical than an apparently low cost practice. Drugs that seem expensive in general practice may save money for the NHS in the long run – this is a very under-researched area. There is still a long way to go.

5 Generic prescribing

Morgan P Feely

Background

Three different types of name may be used to describe a medicinal drug: the full chemical name, the approved (generic, official, non-proprietary) name or a proprietary (brand) name. Similarly, a product containing a combination of drugs may be described by an approved name or a proprietary name, e.g. co-amilofruse or (one of several brands) Frumil®. The chemical name of a drug is usually very long, and, thus, unsuitable for use in prescribing. The term **generic prescribing** is widely used and accepted to describe the prescribing of drugs by their approved names, as opposed to their proprietary names. Strictly speaking, this is actually a misuse of the term generic (derived from latin, genea), already used to describe a genus or class of object; in this case barbiturate would be a true generic name while phenobarbitone, a specific barbiturate, would not.

When a drug is new and still protected by patents usually only one, proprietary, preparation is available. In some cases, as a result of commercial agreements, a drug still protected by patent may be marketed by two different firms, under two different proprietary names (e.g. lisinopril as Carace® and Zestril®). When the patent expires a number of different preparations, including alternative proprietary formulations and/or formulations without a proprietary name, may become available. The latter are often referred as generic drugs or 'generics'. The term 'generic drugs' has also been said to describe 'interchangeable multisource pharmaceutical products'.

Most hospitals in the UK have a policy that permits **generic substitution**. Whether the hospital doctor writes a proprietary name or the approved name, the formulation, or one of the formulations, stocked by the pharmacy is dispensed; this may be a proprietary formulation or a 'generic' without a proprietary name. Some states, including states in the USA, permit community pharmacists to make generic substitutions, although there may be a form of words which the prescriber can write on the prescription to indicate that this is unacceptable. In the United Kingdom community pharmacists are in breach of their terms of service if the prescriber writes a proprietary name but they dispense some other formulation. Where the prescriber uses the generic name the pharmacist may dispense the cheapest acceptable formulation available.

There are advantages and disadvantages to the prescribing of drugs by their generic names; the challenge in writing this chapter is to produce a balanced view regarding these advantages and disadvantages. While generic versions of parenteral preparations of many drugs are available, most of the controversy about generic prescribing has focused on oral formulations and this chapter will have a similar emphasis.

The main issues

There are two major issues, cost and safety. Where the pharmacist is able to dispense the cheapest acceptable formulation there are often, but not always, worthwhile savings to be had in the drug budget. The use of generics, or/and generic prescribing, has been advocated for years in many Western countries largely for economic reasons. In USA the use of generics rose from 10% in 1975 to 21% by 1986. In the latest figures for prescribing by general practitioners in England (December 1994) 54% of prescriptions were generic.

There is a theoretical possibility (and it is mostly just theoretical) that by failing to specify a particular formulation the prescriber leaves the patient open to the possibility (risk) of getting a product that is in some way unsuitable, or less suitable, for the purpose intended. The preparation dispensed could (theoretically):

- fail to contain, or contain much too little or much too much of, the drug in question

- contain some impurity that is toxic

- have a constituent, for example an excipient, that, while not toxic for most patients, induces an allergic reaction in the patient in question

- lack **bioequivalence** with the formulation of the same drug that the patient has been taking prior to getting this prescription.

In practice, since no pharmacist should dispense other than an approved formulation, the possibility of the first or second of these things occurring in the UK nowadays is extremely remote, and it is the third and fourth possibilities, particularly the latter, which sometimes cause the problems. The first drug safety legislation in the United States followed an episode in the 1930s when the use of diethylene glycol as a solvent for sulphanilamide (elixir) caused over 50 deaths.

Bioequivalence

The equivalence of pharmaceutical products can be established at several different levels: chemical equivalence, pharmaceutical equivalence, bioequivalence and therapeutic equivalence. Definitions for all of these are provided in the review by Gleiter and Gundert-Remy referenced at the end of the chapter. The **bioavailability** of a drug is defined as 'the rate and extent to which the active substance (therapeutic moiety) is absorbed from a pharmaceutical form and becomes available at the site of action'. Medicinal products are bioequivalent 'if they are pharmaceutical equivalents (contain the same amount of the same active substance(s) in the same dosage form(s)) and their bioavailabilities after administration in the same (molar) doses are similar to such an extent that their effects, with respect of both efficacy and safety, will be essentially the same'. This latter definition is attributed to the Committee for Proprietary Medicinal Products (CPMP) of the European Community. Only **therapeutic equivalence** guarantees a comparable therapeutic effect after exchanging one brand for another. The issue thus becomes – what level or standard of bioequivalence testing assures therapeutic equivalence?

As a result of past problems (mentioned in the following section) resulting from lack of bioequivalence between brands, and sometimes within brands after a change in the production process, regulatory authorities, such as the FDA, have developed rules/guidelines for testing bioavailability and bioequivalence. A major feature of such testing consists of comparing the difference in areas under the plasma concentration–time curve (AUC) between original brand and new (generic) preparation. For example, EC guidelines for the AUC ratio require that the 90% confidence interval should lie within a range of 0.80 to 1.25. In most cases, such 'rules' have been set arbitrarily, and they can be varied. The ranges may be tightened for drugs with a narrow therapeutic 'window'. Unfortunately, when additional preparations are licensed, information as to the 'yardstick' that was applied is not readily available to prescribers; as far as can be ascertained, in the UK, a tighter range has been applied only to phenytoin.

Two additional points from the review of bioequivalence and drug toxicity by Gleiter and Gundert-Remy are worth highlighting.

1 They state that, to their knowledge, in recent years, following advances in standardizing the testing of bioavailability and bioequivalence there have been no (new) reports of clinical consequence of bioinequivalence.

2   They point out that the European Community guidelines on testing do
not require that the excipients (of different 'brands') need to be identical,
nor do they define the degree of impurity that is allowed.

Past problems due to bioinequivalence

Many of the documented cases of bioinequivalence giving rise to adverse
clinical outcomes have involved, not surprisingly, drugs with a narrow
therapeutic range (window), such as phenytoin, digoxin and carbamazepine.
In the late 1960s, in Australia, calcium sulphate dihydrate was replaced by
lactose as an excipient in a phenytoin preparation. An unexpected increase in
(oral) bioavailability resulted and many patients who had been stabilized on
the former preparation developed evidence of intoxication.

Phenytoin is an extreme example: not only has it a narrow therapeutic
range but saturable metabolism acts as a multiplier of any change in (dose
or) bioavailability. In one patient a 55% change in blood level after a 7%
change in dose was documented. Therefore, it is not difficult to envisage
that a 3 or 4% change in bioavailability could produce sufficient change
in blood level to give rise to intoxication (or therapeutic failure). I believe
that in the early 1980s the manufacturer of one well known phenytoin brand
had difficulty demonstrating to the regulatory authority that there was
consistency between batches of the drug, and indeed that, in effect, 2×50
was the same as 100! For some drugs it may be necessary that bioequivalence
studies are done at steady state and in patients with blood levels within
the therapeutic range. It may be the case that, for some drugs with a
narrow therapeutic range, tight(er) ranges need to be set in relation to the
AUC ratio.

Where drugs have a narrow therapeutic window either intoxication or
lack of effect may result from bioinequivalence. In separate reports, both of
these occurrences have been reported with drugs such as digoxin and
carbamazepine. Other drugs where bioinequivalence has been reported to
cause lack of effect include oxytetracycline and glibenclamide.

In some cases, lack of therapeutic equivalence may be due to an excipient
or impurity causing an 'allergic' response. Erythema multiforme developing
after a patient was switched from Tegretol® to a generic preparation has
been reported. One patient had a skin complaint attributed (correctly) to an
excipient in Epilim®. The widely publicized problem of eosinophilia myalgia
syndrome following tryptophan ingestion has been attributed to an impurity.
Similarly, during the illicit production of a 'designer' opiate in California, a
contaminant, known as MPTP, led to Parkinsonism.

Modified release preparations

The *British National Formulary* has adopted the term 'modified release' (m/r) to cover these products; some were previously described by terms such as 'controlled release' or 'sustained release' (SR). In appropriate circumstances, they may aid compliance, improve efficacy and/or reduce side effects. In relation to this chapter, there are two points to remember.

1 Modified release preparations should be prescribed by brand name.

Failure to do so is likely to have adverse consequences for patients taking drugs with a narrow therapeutic range. The Medicines Control Agency recommends prescribing by brand name in the case of these products.

2 Standard and modified release formulations are not therapeutic equivalents.

Used appropriately, modified release preparations may often have a therapeutic advantage (as summarized above–for details see the review mentioned at the end of this chapter) but they can be disadvantageous. For example, using Tegretol Retard® for new patients may aid compliance and reduce the incidence of side effects, but switching a patient who has been stabilized on the standard formulation to the modified release may result in an increase in seizures. It needs to be pointed out too that there is little, if any, 'compliance gain' with once a day compared with twice a day, and modified release preparations are nearly always more expensive.

Other considerations

Prescribing by approved name is believed to be helpful in increasing the doctor's awareness of what is actually in his/her prescription. Factors favouring the use of proprietary names include ease of remembering some proprietary names (e.g. Piriton® is easier than chlorpheniramine maleate) and continuity of treatment in terms of its appearance to the patient.

The author believes that the first and last of these have been under-investigated and may be important. In a study of the accuracy of doctors' (hospital and GPs) records of their patients' current drug therapy which was carried out in Leeds about ten years ago, a few examples of patients taking two versions of the same drug, (e.g. Lanoxin® and digoxin) were found. This would not have happened if the doctors had been more aware of their prescriptions and/or both items dispensed had not been identical in appearance. As someone with a major interest in compliance, the author is convinced that lack of continuity in the appearance of the medicine dispensed to the patient is sometimes an important factor in 'pill muddle'.

Conclusion

Doctors should prescribe generically in most instances: a high level of generic prescribing is a desirable goal, but we should neither seek nor expect to attain 100%.

Generic prescribing (substitution) should be avoided in the following circumstances:

1   when prescribing modified release preparations

2   where drugs have narrow therapeutic range (e.g. phenytoin, carbamazepine, lithium, theophylline) and patients have already been stabilized on a particular brand

3   where it appears that a change in formulation has previously appeared to produce an adverse reaction, such as a drug rash.

In the author's view, the possibility of 'pill muddle' is not a reason for avoiding generic prescribing, except in very rare instances, but doctors and (especially) pharmacists need to be more alert to this problem, and guard against it by explanation to the patients (and sometimes the relatives too).

Further reading

Anon. (1994/95) Modified Release Preparations. *Medicines Resource,* **20:** 75–8.
Gleiter C H and Gundert-Remy V. (1994) Bioinequivalence and Drug Toxicity: How great is the problem and what can be done? *Drug Safety,* **11**(1): 1–6.

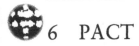

6 PACT

John J Ferguson

The Prescription Pricing Authority (PPA) is a special health authority within the NHS in England which can trace its origins back to 1913. It currently processes 458 million prescription items annually and the number of prescriptions has been rising by 4% per annum. The total cash value is over £3.4 billion per annum, which is approximately 10% of the total expenditure of the NHS in England.

The National Insurance Act, introduced by Lloyd George in 1911, gave low-paid workers the right to a consultation with their doctor and the necessary medicines from a pharmacist free of charge. Initially chemists dispensed the medicine, priced their own prescriptions, and billed the local medical committee for the cost of the medicines they had supplied under this scheme. Within a couple of years, this system was thought to be unsatisfactory, and pricing was transferred to local pricing bureaux. Over the next 60 years there was little change in the process of manual pricing of ever-increasing numbers of the prescriptions and the reimbursement of pharmacists.

In 1976, Dr R Tricker, Director of the Oxford Centre for Management Studies, was invited by the Secretary of State for Social Services to undertake a fundamental inquiry into the functions, organization and constitution of the PPA. The decision to hold the inquiry was promoted by, first, concern over the delays in paying the accounts of chemist contractors and dispensing doctors, and, secondly, difficulties in obtaining information about prescribing patterns which was urgently needed to assit in tackling the problem of the cost of the pharmaceutical services. He clearly identified that the short-term problems of prescription processing could be overcome in the long term only by computerization which, in turn, would provide an information feedback system to GPs and health authorities on patterns of prescribing.

The first computerized information system was based on the manual PD2/PD8 system which was used by only a small number of practitioners. Experience with this system led to the development of a more informative and selective information system, prescribing analysis and cost (PACT). To ensure that the PACT system met the needs of GPs, a user group with members from the Department of Health, Prescription Pricing Authority, General Medical Services Committee, Royal College of General Practitioners, Royal Pharmaceutical Society and Society of FPS Administrators was set up. It was decided to produce a system that would provide general practitioners with well-presented, timely and frequent information. In order to ensure that users were not swamped with information, the system was designed to present the information at three different levels, depending on the needs of the GPs.

The PACT system was implemented in August 1988 and approximately every three months each GP received a summary of his or her prescribing for the previous quarter in the form of an automatic level I report. Level II reports highlighted the areas of prescribing where the major costs were incurred and were 'remedial' in the sense that they were sent automatically to GPs whose overall prescribing costs had exceeded a predetermined threshold; they were also available on request. Level III reports were issued only at the request of individual practitioners, as they contained a full catalogue of all the prescriptions issued during the quarter and provided a level of detail which was useful to those interested in self-audit of their prescribing or in the development of formularies or practice protocols.

The Leeds PACT pilot scheme demonstrated that substantial savings in the drug budget could be achieved using PACT, by generic prescribing, therapeutic substitution and reducing inappropriate prescribing. Spencer and van Zwanenberg recognized that PACT was a vast improvement over the PD8 scheme, especially in the presentation of data, but that it had limitations as it did not identify clinical factors or repeat prescribing. Within a year of the introduction of PACT and the receipt by GPs of details of their prescribing, the PPA was able to show that the number of high-spending doctors was decreasing, suggesting that feedback works.

In 1991 the NHS Management Executive called for a more integrated approach to the planning, management and delivery of primary and secondary health care, including pharmaceutical services, and stated that the rational effective use of medicines requires pharmacists to work in close collaboration with doctors, nurses and other health and social care professions.

As a result of these changes it was clear that the time had come for the PACT reports to be updated and improved. Extensive consultations were undertaken with the profession and all those interested in prescribing information, and wherever possible, their suggestions were incorporated into the new PACT reports. The first is the standard PACT report, which replaced the PACT level I and level II reports. This report is issued quarterly to all prescribers, health authority professional advisers, and appropriate sections of the NHS Executive and the Department of Health. The PACT standard report (first issued in August 1994) is an eight page A4 landscape report including a four page article in the centre of the report. The report is sequenced so that each page provides an increased level of detail. These were designed to be high quality, user-friendly reports with additional features such as the practice's top 20 drugs, generic prescribing and the proportion of new drugs included for the first time. Standard PACT reports contain, within a standard format, much individual practice-specific prescribing information. The previous streaming of reports has been discontinued: they are now sent simultaneously to all GPs in England every three months towards the end of February, May, August and November. At the end of each quarter, in the course of ten working days, the PPA produces some 29 000 individual prescribing reports off its mainframe information computer, through a high-speed laser printer. Scotland, Wales and Northern Ireland have their own pricing departments and issue their own prescribing reports.

The important features of these new PACT reports are now highlighted using a sample report along with suggestions as to how the information can be used to monitor prescribing.

Page one

Page one (Figure 6.1, page 53) shows a simple bar chart of the practice's prescribing costs for the quarter compared with the FHSA equivalent (average) and the national equivalent (average). The FHSA equivalent is based on the actual figures for the local FHSA adjusted to create an imaginary practice with the same proportion of patients aged 65 years and over. The national equivalent is created in the same way.

These equivalents allow practices to see how their prescribing compares with other practices in the FHSA or nationally. The individual GP's prescribing costs are also shown. Figures are given to show how these various costs have changed from the previous year.

Discussion point

- If your practice's costs are above or below the local or national equivalent, you may want to find out why.

Page two

On page two (Figure 6.2) the practice prescribing costs (and FHSA equivalents) are broken down into the national top six *BNF* therapeutic areas: currently, in order, gastro-intestinal, cardiovascular, respiratory, central nervous system, endocrine, musculoskeletal and joint diseases, and other.

Alongside the costs in each therapeutic area for the first time is a figure giving the percentage of the prescribing costs in each area that is due to new drugs. Drugs are defined as 'new' for three years after their introduction. (Only new drugs that carry the CSM's black triangle symbol are included.)

Also on this page is a list of the 20 leading-cost drugs in the practice giving the number of prescriptions, their total cost, the percentage of the practice total and the change from last year. In addition, brand-name drugs in the list are flagged with a 'G' if a generic preparation is available.

Discussion points

- The bar chart on page two can indicate therapeutic areas where costs are different from the local equivalent. Are there any reasons for these differences?

- The top 20 leading-cost drugs highlight individual drugs that are costing the practice a lot of money. Is the prescribing of these drugs appropriate?

- Where branded products in this list are marked with a 'G' it may be worth finding out how much may be saved by switching to the generic.

Page three

This page concentrates on the number of items prescribed rather than costs (Figure 6.3). An item is equivalent to each order for a product written on an FP10, but the size of an item (amount prescribed) is not considered. The chart shows:

- the number of items prescribed by the practice compared with FHSA and national equivalents

- the percentage of items written generically

- the percentage actually dispensed generically.

These figures are different because prescriptions may be written generically for products that are not available as a generic preparation and therefore the brand is dispensed. The number of items prescribed is then broken down into the various therapeutic areas. The introduction of patient treatment packs will mean that an item will, in future, be more clearly defined.

Discussion points

- How does your practice compare with the FHSA and national equivalent?

- What is the difference between the generic prescribing percentage and the dispensed-generically percentage?

● Does the practice have a policy on generic prescribing?

Page four

Page four (Figure 6.4) combines the elements of the earlier data to provide details of the average cost per item for the practice compared to the FHSA and national equivalents. The average costs per item are also shown in each of the therapeutic areas.

The average cost per item will depend largely on the amount prescribed on each prescription and may well reflect practice policy on repeat prescribing. If costs per item vary widely from the averages you may want to find out why.

Page five

Six graphs on page five (Figure 6.5) show the changes in practice prescribing costs and FHSA equivalents over the last eight quarters in the six main therapeutic areas, demonstrating:

● seasonal variation

● how prescribing policy changes affect costs, e.g. increased use of anti-inflammatories in asthma

● whether the practice spending is converging or diverging from local patterns of prescribing.

Pages six and seven

An extensive table on pages six and seven (Figures 6.6 and 6.7) ranks the practice's own top 40 sections of the BNF in terms of cost. The number of items prescribed in each section is given along with comparisons with the FHSA and the practice's last year figures.

This table allows the practice to identify the therapeutic sections that account for the largest proportion of its spending on drugs. These may be the sections that the practice may wish to concentrate its attention on through the use of the more detailed information available in the prescribing catalogue.

Discussion point

● Is prescribing in the most expensive therapeutic areas rational?

Page eight

Practice details such as list size are carried on the back page together with details of items personally administered or dispensed by the practice (Figure 6.8). If the details are not approximately correct, the comparative percentages calculated in the report will not be of any value. These items are those that attract payment under paragraph 44.5 of the Statement of Fees and Allowances (Red Book). A glossary of terms is also included on this page.

PACT centre pages

There is an insert in the centre of the standard PACT report that is concerned with some important and topical aspects of prescribing in general practice. It is illustrated by national trends in prescribing and looks at the quality issues raised by this aspect of prescribing (Figure 6.9). There is additional practice-specific prescribing feedback related to the topic of the centre pages. The subjects covered so far are asthma and inhalers; diuretics and potassium therapy; depression and antidepressants; hormone replacement therapy; and antibiotics. The editor of this section is the Medical Director of the Prescription Pricing Authority, and there is also a multidisciplinary editorial board.

These new PACT reports have been well received and have generated much spontaneous comment. The editor of the *Drug and Therapeutics Bulletin* thought 'new PACT had impact'. The *British Medical Journal* editorial believed that the 'new PACT reports make the best prescribing data in the world even better'. A GP simply thought is was 'PACT with information'.

The prescribing catalogue

Prescribing catalogues replace the old level III reports and are available only on request. The report provides details of every item prescribed and dispensed by the practice or individual GP. As a result the full report runs to about 100 pages. A prescribing catalogue may be requested for the practice overall, or for individual partners or registrars, or if so desired it may be restricted to one or more individual therapeutic areas.

The first few pages of the report repeat information provided in the standard report and give additional details of prescribing rates. The remainder sets out in detail every item that has been dispensed in the quarter, with the quantity prescribed and the cost. It also sums the total number of tablets/doses prescribed per presentation. The catalogue flags products available generically (GFA), new drugs (N), controlled drugs (CD), CSM monitored drugs (CSM) and borderline substances (BS).

The prescribing catalogue and audit

The prescribing catalogue is by far the more valuable of the two reports if a practice wants to look in detail at its prescribing patterns or to monitor the effects of any changes in prescribing policy. The sheer volume of information provided may be daunting, but the key to success is to tackle it in manageable stages.

Limitations of PACT

PACT data are extremely valuable but, as with any statistical information, they have their limitations and potential pitfalls. GPs need to be aware of these in order to avoid drawing the wrong conclusions and using the data inappropriately.

Comparisons with FHSA and national equivalents

The population characteristics of an individual practice are unique and may vary enormously within one FHSA. Prescribing in any practice is determined in part by the characteristics of the patient population. When comparing prescribing with local and national averages demographic factors need to be borne in mind, as PACT data are not very sensitive to them (see Chapter 4).

Prescribing units

PACT data recognize that elderly patients generally require more prescriptions than patients in other age groups. Thus, for comparative purposes, the patient population is described in terms of prescribing units, or PUs. Under this system, patients of 65 and over count as 3 PUs on the crude basis that they require on average three times as many prescriptions as the under 65s.

The bar charts in the standard PACT report compare each practice with a fictional 'average' or equivalent practice. The figures for this average practice are obtained by dividing the total costs or total number of items in the FHSA in that quarter by the total number of PUs in the FHSA. This gives an average cost or number of items per PU in the FHSA.

These figures are then multiplied by the number of PUs in your practice to give the costs and number of items for a practice of similar size and age profile prescribing at the average rate for the FHSA.

ASTRO-PUs

The Prescribing Research Unit in Leeds has developed a weighting system – the age, sex and temporary resident originated prescribing unit (ASTRO-PU) that takes greater account of the differing prescribing needs of males and females in nine different age bands. It allows more accurate comparisons between practices and is already being used to help calculate prescribing budgets (see Chapter 4).

Practice list size

The prescribing and cost rates given in PACT are based on the practice list size held by the FHSA. While this is fine in areas where the population is stable, prescribing and cost rates may not be accurate where the list size is rapidly changing. Data for individual partners are also based on their personal list size, so unless GPs see only patients registered with them, and use only their own FP10 pads, individual comparisons with practice and other equivalents are of little value.

Cost per item

When looking at cost per item for the practice compared with FHSA and national averages it is important to remember that this figure depends on the quantity of drug prescribed each time. A practice that always prescribes repeat prescriptions for three months will have a higher cost per item than a practice that prescribes one month's treatment. Cost per item should be looked at in conjunction with the number of items prescribed.

Individual GP prescribing

PACT data for individual GPs relate to the prescriptions written on the GP's prescription pad or under that doctor's unique prescriber number. Where one doctor's FP10s are used for repeat prescribing or nurse-requested items or where the registrar uses the trainer's pad, the PACT data are distorted. For audit purposes aggregated practice data should be requested.

Electronic PACT

Professional prescribing advisers need to able to cope with a vast amount of PACT data for their health authority, and so an electronic Management

Services Information System (MSIS) has been developed for them along with the PACTLINE analysis package that was first released in 1992. This provides electronic prescribing information on a monthly basis down to *BNF* chapter and section level. Prescribing patterns and trends can be readily identified, and easily understood graphs and reports can be produced.

FHSA electronic PACT (FEPACT)

FEPACT is the next step in the development of further prescribing information that was started by PACTLINE. It was produced by the PPA to enable professional advisers to obtain prescribing information down to individual drugs, and was implemented in a phased manner between November 1994 and March 1995 to all 90 FHSAs in England. Because of the size of the database, it was impossible to download this information, so FEPACT was developed as a 'client/server' application to allow FHSA advisers to gain access to prescribing information held on the PPA's mainframe information computer. Queries are generated by the individual adviser and may be requested for any number of practices or subsets over a range of time. Trends in drug use are identified by asking the same question on a monthly basis. The system runs under Windows and is designed to interface with the existing PACTLINE system; a user can run both systems under Windows and 'toggle' between them.

General practitioner electronic PACT (GPE PACT)

GPE PACT has been designed as an electronic link system that will provide individual GP practices with their prescribing down to individual drug level on a monthly basis. It will allow GPs to monitor and analyse their own and their partners' prescribing and to compare this with that of the FHSA. The system was developed during 1994 and is currently being piloted with some selected general practices. The analysis package will be able to perform profile, trend and financial analysis and will be of particular interest to fundholding and dispensing practices.

PACT and the future

Prescribing is an important activity in general practice. If we are to understand it better, it may well be that we all need to collect further information about the diagnosis and the patient, either directly or indirectly, through data linkage systems.

The aim at the PPA is to collect and feedback more information electronically, using the NHS information highway. The PPA has already carried out some limited pilot studies of electronic prescribing from health centres and dispensing doctors to test the methods.

Even though the majority of general practices are computerized, it is not believed that GPs and their computing systems are ready for electronic PACT reports. Maybe in five to ten years time all GPs will be so computer literate that PACT reports on paper will be a thing of the past.

Appendix: The PACT Standard Report

PACT

PPA
PRESCRIPTION PRICING AUTHORITY
NHS PRESCRIBING INFORMATION CENTRE

STANDARD REPORT

BNF Version Number 26

QUARTER ENDING DECEMBER 1994

For explanatory notes and practice details, please see back page

PRACTICE PRESCRIBING COSTS

		Change from last year (%)
Your practice	£439,835	11
FHSA equivalent	£490,672	7
National equivalent	£470,908	7
Your own costs	£28,122	19

Your Practice costs are **below** the FHSA equivalent by 10%
Your Practice costs are **below** the national equivalent by 7%

Figure 6.1 Page 1 of *PACT Standard Report*. (Reproduced with permission of the Prescription Pricing Authority. PACT is a registered trade mark of the Prescription Pricing Authority.)

YOUR PRACTICE COSTS BY BNF THERAPEUTIC GROUP

	Practice costs / FHSA equivalent	Comparison with FHSA (%)	Change from last year (%) Practice	FHSA	% new drugs
Gastro-Intestinal System	£67,160 / £79,953	−16	10	8	8
Cardiovascular System	£60,564 / £85,657	−29	2	6	1
Respiratory System	£48,068 / £56,039	−14	10	5	7
Central Nervous System	£57,470 / £56,529	2	7	14	13
Endocrine System	£33,120 / £36,807	−10	20	15	12
Musculoskeletal & Joint Diseases	£23,790 / £25,009	−5	1	−9	1
All other	£149,663 / £150,678	−1	18	8	2

THE TWENTY LEADING COST DRUGS IN YOUR PRACTICE
These drugs represent 32.7% of your total practice cost. G: generic form available

Drug	Total cost (£)	% practice total	Change from last year (%)	No. of items
1: Omeprazole	24,489	5.6	27	422
2: Ranitidine	18,854	4.3	−16	460
3: Fluozone	8,987	2.0	0	1,735
4: Becotide G	8,448	1.9	−27	564
5: Captopril	7,388	1.7	10	323
6: Fluoxetine HCL	7,326	1.7	229	266
7: Diclofenac Sod (Systemic)	6,748	1.5	164	488
8: Beclometh Diprop (Ihn)	6,261	1.4	186	493
9: Dressing and Dressing Packs	5,776	1.3	46	360
10: Havrix	5,507	1.3	255	261

Drug	Total cost (£)	% practice total	Change from last year (%)	No. of items
11: Nifedipine	5,379	1.2	22	349
12: Minocin G	5,153	1.2	−16	153
13: Co-Amoxiclav	4,707	1.1	492	746
14: Two Piece Ostomy Systems	4,458	1.0	−3	34
15: Colostomy Bags	4,195	1.0		34
16: Paroxetine HCL	4,066	0.9	60	135
17: Lisinopril	4,053	0.9	23	141
18: Cefactor	3,913	0.9	28	451
19: Femodene	3,877	0.9	−10	388
20: Lansoprazole	3,742	0.9	0	84

Figure 6.2 Page 2 of PACT *Standard Report.*

THE NUMBER OF ITEMS YOUR PRACTICE PRESCRIBES

		Change from last year (%)	Prescribed generically (%)	Dispensed generically (%)
Your practice	51,746	5	58	51
FHSA equivalent	62,749	1	53	47
National equivalent	62,691	0	52	46
Your own prescribing	3,927	7	67	62

The number of items your Practice prescribed is **below** the FHSA equivalent by **18%**
The number of items your Practice prescribed is **below** the national equivalent by **17%**

PRESCRIBING BY BNF THERAPEUTIC GROUP IN YOUR PRACTICE

No. of items prescribed			Comparison with FIISA (%)	Change from last year (%)		Dispensed generically (%)
	Practice	FHSA equivalent		Practice	FIISA	
Gatro-Intestinal System	3,816	5,443	−30	1	2	46
Cardiovascular System	7,463	12,002	−38	5	5	74
Respiratory System	5,567	5,464	2	6	0	43
Central Nervous System	8,965	10,861	−17	4	2	72
Endocrine System	3,065	3,748	−18	10	4	53
Musculoskeletal & Joint Diseases	2,916	3,250	−10	4	−1	55
All other	19,954	21,981	−9	5	0	37

Figure 6.3 Page 3 of PACT *Standard Report.*

AVERAGE COST PER ITEM

		Change from last year (%)
Your practice	£8.50	6
FHSA equivalent	£7.82	6
National equivalent	£7.51	7
Your own average cost	£7.16	11

The average cost of items prescribed by your Practice is **above** the FHSA equivalent by **9%**
The average cost of items prescribed by your Practice is **above** the national equivalent by **13%**

THE AVERAGE COST BY BNF THERAPEUTIC GROUP IN YOUR PRACTICE

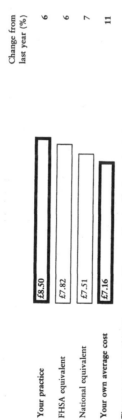

	Your practice		Comparison with FHSA (%)	Change from last year (%) Practice	FHSA
	FHSA equivalent				
Gastro-Intestinal System	£17.60	£14.69	20	9	6
Cardiovascular System	£8.12	£7.14	14	−3	1
Respiratory System	£8.63	£10.26	−16	3	5
Central Nervous System	£6.41	£5.20	23	2	11
Endocrine System	£10.81	£9.82	10	9	11
Musculoskeletal & Joint Diseases	£8.16	£7.70	6	−3	−8
All other	£7.50	£6.85	9	12	8

Figure 6.4 Page 4 of PACT *Standard Report.*

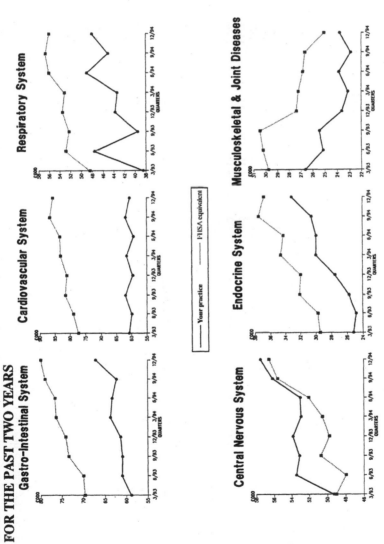

YOUR TOTAL PRACTICE PRESCRIBING COSTS BY BNF THERAPEUTIC GROUP FOR THE PAST TWO YEARS

Figure 6.5 Page 5 of PACT *Standard Report.*

YOUR PRACTICE'S TOP 40 BNF SECTIONS BY COST

Items and costs by section

Ranking			£	Costs Compared with		No.	Items Compared with	
				FHSA (%)	Last year (%)		FHSA (%)	Last year (%)
34	1.2	Antispasmod & Other Drugs Alt Gut Motility	3,332	4	16	406	22	1
1	1.3	Ulcer-Healing Drugs	50,955	-14	9	1,179	-30	8
30	1.5	Treatment of Chronic Diarrhoeas	3,804	7	29	136	7	12
28	1.6	Laxatives	4,116	-44	12	1,076	-37	6
15	2.2	Diuretics	6,773	-18	-9	2,164	-36	1
14	2.4	Beta-Adrenoceptor Blocking Drugs	8,723	-22	-5	1,301	-28	6
4	2.5	Antihypertensive Therapy	21,635	-25	14	1,006	-37	12
8	2.6	Nitrates/Vasodilators/Ca Chann Blockers	17,632	-39	-3	1,499	-43	-6
25	2.12	Lipid-Lowering Drugs	4,221	-24	4	126	-40	21
7	3.1	Bronchodilators	18,135	-17	8	2,980	0	5
3	2.2	Corticosteroids	23,919	-17	4	1,363	-5	8
36	4.1	Hypnotics And Anxiolytics	3,115	-2	73	1,966	-13	6
33	4.2	Drugs Used in Psychoses & Rel. Disorders	3,390	-18	76	395	-41	0
6	4.3	Antidepressent Drugs	20,071	24	24	1,576	-9	18
35	4.6	Drugs Used in Nausea and Vertigo	3,131	-3	6	544	-13	-7
10	4.7	Analgesics	15,902	-6	-8	3,475	-21	1
20	4.8	Antiepileptics	5,734	-7	4	614	-15	-5
21	4.9	Drugs Used in Park'ism/Related Disorders	5,634	-11	25	266	-32	-1
2	5.1	Antibacterial Drugs	33,905	68	20	5,790	12	-6
32	5.2	Antifungal Drugs	3,492	33	0	209	35	-3

Figure 6.6 Page 6 of *PACT Standard Report.*

11	6.1	Drugs used in Diabetes	13,233	0	13	1,028	−14	1
12	6.4	Sex Hormones	12,744	−18	22	712	−17	21
31	6.5	Hypothalamic & Pituitary Hormones & Antioest	3,600	−2	34	36	−8	−14
13	7.3	Contraceptives	12,177	58	9	1,623	57	7
22	8.2	Drugs Affecting The Immune Response	4,775	−15	−23	71	−9	−4
17	8.3	Sex Hormes & Antah In Malig Disease	6,498	−30	41	121	−50	0
16	9.4	Oral Nutrition	6,549	−5	61	408	10	65
5	10.1	Drugs Used in Rheumatic Diseases & Gout	20,566	−3	3	2,430	−10	5
39	10.3	Drugs For Relief of Soft-Tissue Inflamm	2,476	−17	−16	406	−14	−8
37	11.6	Treatment of Glaucoma	2,789	−37	2	378	−39	−5
38	12.2	Drugs Acting on the Nose	2,523	−13	5	472	−2	15
40	13.2	Emollient & Barrier Preparations	2,445	−23	44	700	−16	36
23	13.4	Topical Corticosteroids	4,613	3	11	1,548	3	8
18	13.5	Preparations for Eczema and Psoriasis	5,857	36	57	245	12	12
27	13.6	Preparations for Acne	4,162	149	41	408	134	34
29	13.10	Anti-Infective Skin Preparations	3,928	−10	−2	847	−6	19
9	14.4	Vaccines and Antisera	17,383	−18	58	2,358	−33	24
19	20.3	Dressing And Dressing Packs	5,776	−27	46	360	−39	19
26	23.35	Colostomy Bags	4,195	−30	0	34	−19	−11
24	23.94	Two Piece Ostomy Systems	4,458	84	−3	66	69	−14

Figure 6.7 Page 7 of PACT Standard Report.

PRACTICE PROFILE

	Total list size	Patients 65 & over	Temporary residents	No. PUs
Dr WORKLOAD	1,924	463	0	2,850
Practice	27,801	3,809	218	35,419

TOTAL PRESCRIBING ASCRIBED TO YOU

	Items	Cost (£)
Dr WORKLOAD	3,927	28,122
Trainee	–	–
Deputising services for the Practice	5	9

ITEMS PERSONALLY ADMINISTERED OR DISPENSED BY YOUR PRACTICE

	Personally administered		Dispensed	
	This year	Last year	This year	Last year
Practice cost	£16,650	£9,712	n/a	n/a
of total practice cost	3.79%	2,45%	n/a	n/a
No. of items	2,510	2,161	n/a	n/a
Av. cost/item	£6,63	£4,49	n/a	n/a

Overall av. cost/item £8,50   Last year's overall av. cost/item £8,03

Prescribed Generically These figures relate to items prescribed by the approved name, even when a generic is not available.

Dispensed Generically These figures relate to items where a generic is available and the dispenser has been paid for a generic.

Total list size The total number of patients registered with the practice (including temporary residents and over 65s) as last notified by your FHSA.

EXPLANATORY NOTES Please refer to the PACT/TIPS Technical Guide for more detailed explanations.

FHSA Equivalent Throughout this report all figures represent as "FHSA equivalent" are based on the actual figures for the local FHSA adjusted to create an imaginary practice with the same number of PUs s your practice.

National Equivalent Throughout this report all figures represented as "National equivalent" are based in the actual figures for England adjusted to create an imaginary practice with the same number of PUs as this practice.

Figure 6.8 Page 8 of *PACT Standard Report.*

Change from last year	The % change from the equivalent period last year.
Costs	Total Net Ingredient Cost
Prescribing Units (PUs)	Patients under 65 years of age and temporary residents count as one PU. Patientnd aged 65 or over count as three.
Trainee	These figures represent all prescribing on your prescription forms that have been marked with a D in red ink.
Deputising Services	These figures represent all prescribing by deputising doctors who have used prescription pads stamped with L and specified the senior partner number of your practice.
Therapeutic Groups	The six therapeutic groups listed as those which incurred the highest costs in England from April 1993 to March 1994. The terrm "All other" includes preparations, dressings and appliances.
New Drugs	For the purposes of PACT®, drugs are classified as new for a period of three years after the receipt by the PPA of the first prescription for a black triangle drug (CSM monitored)
Leading Cost Drugs	These drugs, using the names by which they were presented, are those which contributed the most to your costs. All presentations are added together to obtain the figure for each drug. Drugs you have prescribed using a proprietary name and for which a generic form is available, are identified by the letter G.
Personally Administered	Items prescribed and administered by you or a member of your practice team and which attract payments under para 44.5 of the Statement of Fees and Allowances (Red Book).
Dispensed	Items dispensed by a dispensing practice including any personally administered items.
Temporary Residents	The list/size shown for temporary residents is based on the same quarter of the previous year and is included in the total list size.

For more information contact: Help Desk, Prescribing Pricing Authority, Block B, Scottish Life House, Archbold Terrace, Jesmond, Newcastle-upon-Tyne NE2 1DB. Tel: (0191) 2810766 Fax: (0191) 2813628

In the near future you will receive request slips which will allow you to request full details of your prescribing in the form of a prescribing catalogue.

Figure 6.8 contd.

Snr Partner: Dr WORKLOAD
47 BRONCHODILATOR WAY

TREATMENT OF DEPRESSION

	Practice	FHSA equivalent
	Practice Items (%)		
	Practice costs (%)		
Tricyclics (Old)	21.4%	337	592
	3.0%	£602	£1,126
Tricyclics (New and Related)	36.0%	568	683
	16.8%	£3,368	£4,077
SSRIs	38.3%	604	385
	76.1%	£15,271	£10,364
MAOIs	2.7%	42	19
	3.2%	£634	£264
Compound Anti-depressants	1.6%	25	53
	1.0%	£196	£322

Figure 6.9 PACT *Standard Report* article on depression and antidepressants.

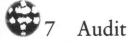 7 Audit

Jacqueline V Jolleys

Audit defined

There are many variations on the definition of audit but all have in common the notion that actual performance is compared to desired standards.

> 'Prescribing audit is the attempt to improve the quality of prescribing by measuring the performance of those providing the service, by considering the performance in relation to desired standards, and by improving on this performance'.

The aims of prescribing audit

Prescribing audit can help the practice improve its prescribing. Good or rational prescribing is characteristically effective, safe, appropriate and economic. Encompassed within this overall aim are the concepts of treating the cause of the condition, where possible avoiding polypharmacy, using drugs with which you are familiar, considering potential drug interactions and monitoring compliance as well as any drug interactions.

The benefits and constraints of prescribing audit

When practices are first considering whether or not to audit prescribing they may at first be put off by the obvious constraint – the considerable time needed for planning, organizing and conducting the work. This may reduce some of the time available for patient care, but the benefits come in terms of quality: patient care may be improved through better control of the clinical condition and early prevention of complications. At the same time, audit forces you to keep your knowledge of therapeutics up to date, promotes effective team working when audit becomes a practice activity, and leads to the development of consistent practice prescribing policies so that patients can no longer play the partners off against each other. In any case, audit does not have to be a constant activity but can be done intermittently to coincide with times when the practice is least busy.

Examples of prescribing audit

The following are some examples of the many areas that may be audited.

Repeat prescribing audit

Repeat prescribing is a relatively easy area in which to begin, since computerized data are readily available in most practices. Examples of more general areas which a practice may like to audit include the scale of repeat prescribing, repeat prescribing of specific drug groups, the frequency of patient review in surgery, and drug quantities supplied. Any of these may lead to changes in repeat prescribing policies and systems.

Another way in which to audit repeat prescribing is to review prescribing on an individual patient basis. This may include consideration of the appropriateness of medication for the patient's condition and whether the medication is still needed. Additional areas to audit could be: compliance, potential drug interactions, recall interval and monitoring, looking to see how often it is that the doctor with clinical responsibility for the patient signs the prescriptions. The use of a specific drug may be put under scrutiny, with a review of prescribing indications, efficacy, compliance, potential drug interactions, noting any side effects and looking at the patient review interval.

Example: Audit of patients taking lithium salts

Areas to consider for auditing might include:

- is there the correct indication? – mania, hypomania or prevention of mania and depression
- is there continued need?
- is the treatment effective?

- is there potential for drug interaction? – diuretics, NSAIDs, etc., being prescribed concurrently

- is the patient reviewed regularly?

- the incidence of side effects?

- are patients getting their repeat prescriptions at the right intervals?

- are serum levels monitored regularly?

- since bioavailability varies from one product to another (in particular the modified release preparations), is prescribing by brand name?

Review of patients on multiple medication

GPs can decide for themselves what to look at: it may be that all patients receiving three medications or more concurrently are reviewed, or all patients over 75, so that prescribing review becomes part of their health check. The aims of the review will vary – some of the likely ones include:

- effective, appropriate prescribing, reviewing the patient's indications for medication and ensuring that the prescribed medication is appropriate for the patient's condition, age group, etc.

- simplifying the medication regime

- checking compliance

- elimination of incompatible drugs

- avoidance of prescribing error.

Audit of particular classes of drugs

This type of audit is defined and relatively easy to conduct but can yield useful information. Particularly worthwhile examples include peptic ulcer therapy, antidepressants, NSAIDs and benzodiazepines.
The sort of questions posed are:

- is the medication being prescribed as recommended for licensed indications, at licensed dosage?

- are known side effects being monitored?

- are required checks including laboratory investigations being conducted?

- are the practice prescribing guidelines or practice formulary being complied with?

- is there a policy on generic prescribing? Is this being followed?

Example: Audit of medication for gout

Patients who suffer from a particular condition e.g. gout may be identifiable from a disease register. Further patients may be found by reviewing repeat prescriptions of all medications used to treat that particular complaint: Zyloric 100, allopurinol 100, Zyloric 300, allopurinol 300, Hamarin 300, any NSAID used regularly for the condition, and uricosuric drugs. This should give a reasonable estimate of the number of sufferers, so that the practice prevalence can be compared with epidemiological data; the proportion on regular preventative treatment is also worth noting. Diagnostic criteria and the need for regular prophylaxis can be reviewed, and for those patients not on regular treatment, the medical records examined to see the frequency of attacks and whether prophylactic therapy is indicated. Finally, substitution of the brand name products with generic can produce worthwhile savings on costs.

Case-based auditing

Although it sounds threatening, a lot can be learned from examining prescribing problems or failures of treatment to try to identify any management errors or omissions that may have affected the outcome. While investigating the specifics of the case, lessons are learned which, if acted upon, will have wider implications.

Specific applications of audit

Audit is a means by which a practice can **detect underprescribing**. This is important in conditions where taking medication regularly is known to affect the patient's wellbeing as well as the clinical outcome, e.g. asthma, depression, moderate/severe hypertension. With asthma this could entail auditing use of prophylactic drugs and 'relievers', and considering whether their relative use is in line with the British Thoracic Society guidelines. Alternatively, audit might alert the practice to the fact that it has identified, and is treating, fewer sufferers from a particular disease than would be expected from the known prevalence.

It is a means of **detecting over prescribing**. Audit activities can show where repeat medication is being requested too frequently; where more than one pharmacological preparation is prescribed concurrently for the same condition; where medication is being prescribed to counteract the unwanted effect of another drug; or where a patient's repeat medication was not reviewed on receipt of a request from a consultant to prescribe a particular medication – the new medication being added without any consideration of another one being stopped.

Other uses of audit are **the detection of patient compliance problems** such as the selective compliance of a patient who is taking a diuretic and a betablocker for the treatment of hypertension but chooses not to take the diuretic when going out or socialising and thus is only intermittently being adequately medicated.

Patient-initiated over medication may also be audited, to detect the possibility of habituation, as with hypnotics, anxiolytics and analgesics, and other situations where with over use side effects can be problematic i.e. topical eczema corticosteroid preparations.

By auditing a particular aspect of its prescribing the practice can see whether it has amended its prescribing in the light of revised indications, the publication of a warning over prescribing a medication for a particular patient group, or the findings of well-susbstantiated research. In peptic ulcer disease, the practice might want to know how often it uses Helicobacter pylori eradication therapy.

Through prescribing audit the practice can identify those patients who take a **drug that has little therapeutic value** and may often pick up cases where there has been a **prescribing error** e.g. errors of dose, quantity or duration, incompatibility problems and inappropriate indication.

Selecting performance standards for audit

There are few published therapeutic protocols to guide a practice when it is deciding upon the standards it wants to achieve. It will often have to define its own benchmarks against which to monitor performance, and these have to take into account local factors like the morbidity patterns, expectations and beliefs of the population. As well as the general principles of good practice most doctors adopt implicit or explicit criteria for managing common clinical conditions. Standards take the form of the proportion of cases in which these criteria are followed. The proportion may be selected on the basis of consensus opinion or, where applicable, acceptable evidence.

Even going through the motions of audit is likely to enhance the quality of prescribing in a practice, because the staff will become alerted to specific aspects and pitfalls, and the general practitioners will improve their knowledge of therapeutics as a result of the discussions that ensue. Even more benefit occurs when standards are debated and set, audit is conducted and performance is reviewed in terms of those standards. Many GPs get very interested and involved once they begin to examine standards, and agree how and where they want to improve. They find the process intellectually stimulating, educational, and professionally rewarding.

The cyclical nature of audit

A single audit confers limited benefit. The strength of audit is its cyclical nature and the opportunity it presents to recognize, monitor and quantify the effects of changes in a practice stimulated by previous audit activities. The review is thus ongoing, creating in part a continuous quality assurance programme.

The development and monitoring of therapeutic guidelines

Inspired by audit GPs are often moved to develop a clinical protocol for the management of chronic conditions. These define the standards of care and prescribing that the practice wishes to deliver to every patient. Future delivery can then be monitored against the standards charted in the in-house protocol. Guideline development involves a definition of the condition to be treated; agreed criteria for diagnosis; methods of treatment including any life-style advice; defining the point at which medication is needed; defining desirable outcome and finally monitoring and review procedures. Examples of conditions for which therapeutic guidelines are commonly developed include asthma, hypertension, Type II diabetes, depression and indigestion. The choice of drug or the stepwise treatment schedule is made after informed debate about dose, duration of treatment, and the monitoring of the efficacy and side effects of the medication.

Formulary development and utilization

Prescribing audit often leads to development of a formulary as a means of ensuring quality, appropriate, safe and cost-effective prescribing. When its effectiveness is to be evaluated, departures from the formulary and the reasons that the partners give for them, need to be carefully considered.

Conducting prescribing audit using PACT data

The context of increased accountability and restricted resources in disease management places increasing demands on practices to develop effective prescribing policies.

All practices and doctors receive quarterly PACT standard reports, and a PACT prescribing catalogue that details every prescription issued can be ordered, that makes it possible to conduct a thorough review of prescribing, to audit performance, to develop or update a formulary and to develop clinical protocols.

Prescribing audit conducted in terms of cost alone is of limited value, yet it is one of the easiest types of audit to do from PACT data. You may see that you prescribe more cheaply or relatively expensively in comparison with other practices in your area, or this is at least a starting point. There is a notion, apparently fostered by the Department of Health, that low cost prescribers are virtuous and that high cost prescribers need to be restrained. This is an oversimplification. Virtue lies in meeting the needs of the practice population with a proper regard for economy, and these needs vary with the age and level of morbidity of the population. In order to be able to make direct comparisons in terms of relative costing between one practice and another, a weighting system is needed so that the assigned prescribing population takes into account practice demography and morbidity. For prescribing costs overall, the ASTRO-PU weighting system achieves this; for specific therapeutic groups, there are the analagous STAR-PU weightings (Chapter 4). Without these kinds of standardization, external comparisons are likely to be unreliable: PACT data are better at raising questions than at answering them. The trend data now being given are useful for internal comparisons though – since practice patterns over time can be monitored.

The limitations of PACT data are considered in Chapters 4 and 6.

Audit is a practice team activity

Audit is a practice activity ideally involving all staff members in such a way that their particular skills are utilized. As such it promotes good team working, is rewarding and far from onerous. Developments in practice computerization have made it possible to conduct prescribing audit with relatively limited investment in terms of time since most practices have computerized repeat prescribing programmes and a significant proportion of age/sex and morbidity registers.

Conclusion

Prescribing audit affects the wider aspects of clinical care. Although initially it is a separate activity, in time and with some effort it becomes an integral part of clinical practice involving the whole of the practice team. Repeated audit against regularly revised monitoring standards facilitates the development of a prescribing quality assurance programme.

Further reading

Audit Commission. (1994) *A prescription for improvement. Towards more rational prescribing in general practice.* HMSO, London.

Haines A and Hurwitz B. (1992) *Clinical guidelines: Report of a local initiative.* Occasional paper 58, Royal College of General Practitioners, Exeter.

Marinker M (ed). (1990) *Medical Audit and General Practice* (1st edn) BMJ/ MSD Foundation, London.

Pringle M and Bradley C. (1995) *Significant event auditing: a study of the feasibility and potential of care-based auditing in primary medical care.* Occasional paper 70, Royal College of General Practitioners, Exeter.

Royal College of General Practitioners. (1994) *How to develop a practice formulary.* RCGP Publications, Exeter.

8 Repeat prescribing

Arnold Zermansky

Repeat prescriptions are written in steel and concrete and are not easily dismantled or re-modelled.

Michael Balint, 1970

Repeat prescribing is the UK solution to the problem of ensuring continuous supplies of medication to patients on continuing treatment. It avoids the need for the doctor and patient to meet each time the medication is renewed, saving the doctor and the patient a great deal of time.

It is probably the earliest example of delegation of labour in British general practice, and seems to have begun long before most practices had nurses, managers or secretaries, and decades before computers. Exactly how long ago is difficult to ascertain, since it appears fairly sparsely in research. It seems to have developed spontaneously, presumably in response to need, demand or at least convenience of doctor and patient, throughout the whole of the United Kingdom. In its simplest form the receptionist records the details of the patient's request at the reception desk and prepares a prescription, the doctor signs it and the patient collects it. There is still the occasional practice in which this constitutes the entire process, with no attempt to control the issue of repeat drugs, but this is now very unusual. Virtually all practices record every repeat prescription, and computerization has made the cumbersome business of controlling repeats relatively painless. Most prescribing software suites allow the practice to identify over- and even under-users of medication, and to recall patients at preset intervals for review. Since it is essentially a mechanical process it lends itself to such a delegated approach, and the doctor's only contribution is his signature, often dashed off in bulk whilst drinking coffee at the end of morning surgery, before setting out on home visits.

The cost of repeats

The Audit Commission believes that repeat prescribing probably accounts for about two thirds of all items dispensed in England and Wales. This would make the cost of repeats in 1992/3 about £2.4 billion, representing 80% of the total drug costs, and more than half of the total cost of NHS primary medical care. Recent figures are even higher. It is also a rapidly growing cost – prescribing costs rose by about 14% per annum in 1992/3. The number of patients who are on regular repeats is unknown, but may well be half of the population. Within this group will be a much larger proportion of the sick and old, as well as an increasing number of patients on preventative treatment such as hypotensives and lipid lowering drugs.

The benefits of repeat prescriptions

Repeats are to the mutual advantage of both the doctor and patient (Box 8.1). They allow patients to renew their supply of medication with minimum fuss and without the need for a time-consuming, inconvenient and potentially stressful consultation. The doctor also avoids the need to see the patient, freeing him for more useful (or perhaps more pleasurable!) activities. They reduce the likelihood of the patient running out of tablets, and emphasize the need for continuing and uninterrupted treatment. There is a palpable shift of responsibility for the treatment from the doctor to the patient, who is then in charge of his own illness and destiny, and thereby empowered and perhaps emancipated. Devolution of care to the

---

Box 8.1: Who benefits from repeat prescriptions?

The doctor
- saves time
- saves consultations
- encourages continuity of treatment
- shift of responsibility to ancillary staff
- shift of responsibility to patient

The patient
- saves time
- saves consultations
- ensures continuity of supply
- empowerment

The pharmacist
- predictability of need
- continuity of custom

Drug manufacturer
- therapeutic momentum

---

patient requires the patient to understand his illness and its treatment and puts an additional educational burden upon the doctor and his staff. Ultimately it leads to better compliance and more effective treatment. The doctor also delegates monitoring of use of medication to his receptionist, who will look out for over- and under-use as well as recalling the patient for periodic review, involving the doctor only when a clinical decision is needed.

Therapeutic momentum

There is also a benefit for the pharmacist. The patient on an established repeat regimen is likely to attend regularly for a predictable repeat, and this allows planned ordering of stock. This continuity can be described as therapeutic momentum – the tendency for an established repeat medication to remain unchanged for months or even years. It has major implications for drug manufacturers, who have only to establish a body of patients on treatment for a chronic condition to be assured of a long-term income. Therapeutic momentum has several negative implications, however, and these will be considered later.

Drawbacks of repeat prescribing

The total cost of repeat prescriptions, though huge, is not inherently a problem so long as the drugs provided are effective, safe, well-tolerated and appropriate, and the patients' therapeutic needs are valid. It is also important that the health gain justifies the expense. Achieving this ideal is not always easy, and there are any number of confounding factors than can render the process inefficient, ineffective or even dangerous. Box 8.2 lists the hazards of repeat prescribing.

Repeat prescriptions are easier to establish than to stop. The GP is always under pressure to prescribe, from the patient, from the patient's relatives or carers and from his self-image as a healer and his ardent desire to do something to help. He is influenced by the medical and lay media, by the promotional activity of the pharmaceutical industry and not least by hospital specialists. The last-named sometimes seem to have a degree of faith in the value of therapeutic intervention that is not always shared by GPs. It can be difficult – some would say impossible – to ignore the therapeutic advice of a

---

Box 8.2: Hazards of repeat prescribing

For the patient   – adverse drug reactions
                         – interactions
                         – unnecessary treatment
                         – potentiation of sick role
                         – proliferative polypharmacopathy

For the doctor   – complacency
                         – responsibility to review – extra consultations

For the drug company – sealed-off opportunity

For the NHS   – waste of resources

                         – cost of adverse drug reactions

---

consultant, and most recommendations lead to a repeat prescription. Once established, it needs a positive decision by the GP to stop or change a drug, with the attendant risk that the patient's condition may deteriorate, and the certainty of an additional consultation to evaluate the change.

Discharge medication after hospital admission presents a particularly difficult practical problem for the GP. Patients are commonly discharged from hospital with as little as one week's supply of treatment, and a full summary of the patient's admission may take weeks to arrive. The GP has to decide what to do about the patient's medication on the strength of a brief preliminary discharge letter that may contain an overall diagnosis but rarely explains the reasons for each item prescribed or even an indication of how long the treatment should be continued.

Whilst in many situations the answer may be self-evident (e.g. antibiotics until the end of the course; thyroxine indefinitely), the doctor often has to take a view from the little evidence available at the time. The practical options are quite limited. Either the patient has his new medication entered on his repeat medication file, which will mean that it may not be reviewed for many months (even in a practice with an effective review system), or the doctor gives the patient a 'one-off' prescription and arranges to see him for a further review before authorizing repeats. The latter is clearly the preferable option, but it commits doctor and patient to a further consultation, and can be confounded by the patient in the interim asking the receptionist for a repeat and getting a supply of the medication he was taking before the admission. When the patient ultimately sees the GP (or hospital doctor for that matter) the consultation takes place with each party unknowingly having a different perception of the patient's current medication. This in turn can lead to further therapeutic muddle that could border on farce if pills did not have potential for harm.

There are other common variations on this theme, particularly in practices (sadly quite common), in which receptionists are empowered to change a patient's repeat regimen in accord with the discharge letter after a cursory nod by the doctor. Confusion over the names of generic and proprietary medicines can lead to double dosing or even the wrong drug being prescribed. It is also easy for the receptionist (or doctor) to fail to notice a change in strength or dose of an existing drug, leading to the patient's reverting to the previous dosage.

Proliferative polypharmacopathy

Repeat prescription patients are often old and ill. They may be in and out of hospital and have several co-existing diseases. They may accumulate doctors as well as diseases, and be under the care of several specialists at once. Some may have their medication controlled or monitored by nurses, carers and community pharmacists, each of whom may have a slightly different perception of the patient's medication, which in turn differs from that recorded in the GP's records. It is easy for such patients to be prescribed more and more drugs, each for an apparently valid reason, and to end up on a complicated regimen, all the details of which may not be known to any of the participating clinicians. The drugs themselves may have adverse effects that may not be recognized for what they are, or be managed inappropriately, particularly if the patient presents to the 'wrong' doctor. Interactions are increasingly likely with each drug added to the regimen. Sometimes **piggy-back drugs** are prescribed to deal with the adverse effects of previously prescribed medication. Whilst this may occasionally be justifiable if the first drug is essential and there is no better tolerated substitute, piggy-back prescribing often seems to happen by default. The first response to a suspected adverse drug reaction should always be to stop the drug.

This uncontrolled burgeoning of the patient's regimen with attendant adverse effects, interactions, paradoxical effects on coexisting conditions and continuation of unnecessary medication is **proliferative polypharmacopathy**. It is a sinister and preventable iatrogenic disorder caused by lack of respect for the potency of agents that are designed to interfere with metabolism, and failure to recognize that multiple medication multiplies the risk of interactions. Most of all it results from lack of overall therapeutic control. No one is in charge of the patient or his medication. Taking overall responsibility for the patient is the essence of general practice, and the effective GP is always cognisant of the risks of multiple medication.

Comfortable patients

Patients become attached to their medicines. Regardless of the therapeutic effect the pills become part of their daily ritual. They come to regard them as essential for their continued well-being. Patients on anti-hypersensitive medication who were symptom-free before diagnosis often claim to feel well because of their treatment. They may be reluctant to consider whether their medication is actually needed. The fact of continuing medication can reinforce the sick role and actually potentiate the patient's (and carer's) illness-centred behaviour. Drugs can make illnesses last longer.

Balint describes how repeat medication can support the patient without exposing him to the trauma of a consultation or exploration of the psychological background of the illness. The treatment becomes a substitute for diagnosis rather than the result of it. Any attempt to interfere with the treatment threatens the comfortable and comforting arms-length relationship with the doctor, and the patient resists it. This model of the repeat prescription implies that the nature of the drug is of no relevance. It is the fact of the treatment that is important, and getting repeats reflects the patient's ambivalence: needing support, but not too much.

Comfortable prescribers

Repeat prescriptions also comfort prescribers, though not always appropriately. They can induce a degree of complacency in the doctor that is almost as powerful as the hold they have on the patient. It is easy to assume that the patient's well-being is the result of his treatment. Stopping an established treatment is a brave thing to do, especially if there is the possibility that the patient's condition may deteriorate. Not only may the doctor incur the patient's disfavour, but he is also committing himself (and the patient) to one or more follow-up consultations to evaluate the effect of the change. It may be unfair to suggest that doctors and their patients conspire to maintain continuity of medication, since there is seldom the degree of premeditation implied by that verb, but the effect is often as if they had done so.

Sealed-off opportunities

The pharmaceutical companies see established repeats as being so entrenched that they comprise sealed-off opportunities, preventing them from introducing a new product for those patients. This is why some drug companies support educational initiatives to encourage doctors to review their repeats.

Stopping drugs

There is considerable evidence that many repeat drugs can safely be stopped, thereby reducing the cost of treatment as well as the patient's exposure to drugs and their hazards. Reports in the literature include stopping benzodiazepines, digoxin, diuretics, NSAIDs, hypotensive agents and dipyridamole. In other situations a newer treatment may abolish the need for continuing medication, most notably with the eradication of *H. pylori* in peptic ulcer disease. Not all drug withdrawals are painless, though. Some may produce short-term withdrawal symptoms; in other cases the patient may be shown still to require medication. In some situations attempting withdrawal is foolhardy. Each individual case needs careful assessment.

Wasted drugs

There are no reliable statistics on wasted drugs. There are reports from pharmacists about returned drugs that have not been used, either because they were never taken at all or because they were stopped or switched. These drugs probably form only a small proportion of the total waste. The larger part are the drugs that are taken, but do not need to be. Some should not have been started. Some are no longer needed. Some are of doubtful therapeutic value. Some are simply more expensive preparations than is necessary. Not all prescribing waste can be or should be prevented – preventing waste has its costs too – but prescribers should always be aware of the issue.

The need to be organized

GPs often admit to feelings of guilt about repeat prescribing. They are aware that they could reduce both costs and hazards by exercising better control, but they do not know how to achieve this against a background of many (seemingly more urgent) demands upon their time. Sometimes they confound the problem by overcompensating. They set unachievable targets for medication reviews, which can then be conducted only in a perfunctory way that defeats the object.

There are four simple rules for organizing repeats efficiently:

1   Delegate everything that can be delegated

2   Have a clear protocol for each participant including the patient

3   Make maximum use of the computer

4   Be realistic in your expectations of everyone – including yourself.

Efficiency versus control

The rest of this chapter examines how repeats should be organized so as to achieve the best compromise between efficiency of production and of control. There is always a trade-off between the two. Control takes time and delays the production of repeats. But unnecessary or harmful repeats are inefficient in themselves.

Organizing repeat prescribing

Organizing repeat prescribing involves three levels of activity, each the domain of a particular set of skills.

The production of repeats

The production of repeat prescriptions is generally delegated to reception staff. It is probably best done by a dedicated person who will become

Table 8.1: Domains and skills of the components of a repeat prescribing system.

Activity	Domain	Skills needed
Production	Receptionist	Interpersonal Keyboard accuracy Precision
Control	Practice Manager	Organizational Person management Meticulousness
Initiation Authorization Review	Doctor	Clinical Therapeutics Precision

familiar with the patients and the games they play, the doctors and their behaviours, and the practice protocol for repeats. The most important skill is precision. The receptionist turns up the patient's repeat prescription screen on the computer and selects the drugs that have been requested. If the drugs are requested too soon (or too late) the doctor will need to be informed. If the patient's review interval has expired, the patient may need to be recalled to see the doctor. If the requested drug is not authorized the prescription is not prepared and the doctor is informed. The selected prescriptions are printed out for the appropriate doctor to sign. If there is a query, the prescription is attached to the patient's records with a note of the problem. After signing, the prescription is given to the patient together with any message from the doctor. Patients who overuse their medication or are due for review may need tactful handling to get them to see the doctor. Nearly all practices manage to produce their repeats quickly and efficiently, though some seem to make life hard for themselves by unnecessary duplication of records. Whilst it is important that manual records have an up-to-date list of the patient's current therapy in case the patient is seen without the computer (at home for example), there is little to be gained by recording each issue in the paper record.

Control of repeats

This is the domain of the practice manager, whose responsibility it is to ensure that safe, effective and efficient systems are in place, and also that staff and doctors follow them.

Controlling repeats without a computer is possible but quite laborious. It is infinitely better than failing to control repeats in spite of a computer. There are still a few computer systems around which do not allow the patient to be given a review date, and some which do not warn the prescriber of over- or under-use. Any practice that has such a system should consider an upgrade for this reason alone. Failing to control repeats is dangerous and probably negligent.

The essentials of a control system are as follows.

1 No repeats without initial authorization

Authorization is the doctor's role. The system must ensure that no one can bypass this essential process. Even hospital-initiated drugs require authorization by the GP.

2 Review warning

The signing doctor must be informed when a review is due. Seriously over-due review dates should block prescribing without further authorization.

3 Compliance warning

Patients who are over- or under-using medication (as measured by the number of doses prescribed and the time interval between prescriptions) should be readily identified, preferably by an on-screen warning, and the fact passed to the prescriber.

4 An updated drug list for each patient

The patient or his carer should have a printed list of his current medication. This can be presented by the patient to any other doctor (or dentist, etc.) who treats him.

5 An updated drug list in the patient's paper records

This is necessary when patients are seen at home (or in a room without a computer screen).

6 A record of each issue

The computer record should suffice.

7 A mechanism for handling hospital discharge medication

This is a critical moment! The details of how these are to be achieved should form a written **practice prescribing protocol** with a separate section for each participant.

Initiation, authorization and review

- *Use review dates for the patient*
  Use review dates for the patient, not the number of issues for each drug. Most computer software allows the prescriber to set a number of authorized issues for each drug. This can mean that a patient on six drugs has six recalls for review in whatever period is chosen – they will not coincide for long because items always get out of kilter. It is far simpler to give the patient a review date, and clinically sounder to review the whole person and his treatment than one drug in isolation.

- *Set long review intervals*
  If the review intervals are too short, the workload of reviewing prescriptions becomes impossible. Twelve months is soon enough for most treatments. Remember that many patients will have been seen in the interval, so check the records before recalling the patient. The review interval is just a backstop.

- *Prescribe in multiples of 28 days*
  The prescription will be due for renewal on the same day of the week every time.

- *Prescribe for two months at a time*
  It halves your workload.

Initiation, authorization and review are the domain of the doctor. They are essentially a series of decisions as to whether the prescription is necessary and appropriate at each stage.

Initiating a repeat

It hardly needs saying that no drug should be prescribed unless it is appropriate and necessary. Nonetheless, it is quite easy not to consider whether the patient would be better served by a non-drug treatment, or indeed no treatment at all. If drug treatment is chosen, it should be effective, acceptable to the patient and well-tolerated. It should not interact adversely with other current medication. It should also be the least expensive preparation that will satisfy these requirements. Whilst it should be possible to select the most appropriate drug in advance, the prescriber will know only in retrospect that the choice was right – hence the need to review the patient at least once before conferring repeat prescription status and entering the drug on the patient's repeat file. *Is the drug really necessary?*

Authorization

This should take place when the prescriber is satisfied:

- that the drug is effective
- that the drug is still needed
- that the patient is taking his medication properly
- that there are no important adverse effects.

It is important to look for **objective evidence of efficacy.** Patients like to please their doctors and often report a benefit that evaporates on more specific enquiry. Ask the patient for details of how the symptoms have improved. Try to **measure improvement,** preferably by some objective criterion (such as blood pressure, fructosamine, peak flow, weight etc.). In the case of inherently subjective symptoms such as pain, it is often useful for the patient to keep a diary, measuring the symptom on (say) a five point scale. Never assume that any improvement is acutally due to the medication. Lots of things get better on their own. Adopt a critical frame of mind. *Is the drug really working?*

Even if the patient has improved as a result of treatment, it does not follow that the treatment will be required indefinitely. In many situations treatment can be stopped to see whether symptoms recur. In others a further limited period of treatment may be necessary. *Is the drug still needed?*

Compliance with treatment cannot be assumed. Check that the patient is taking his medication in the correct dosage by the correct route. Inhaler technique should be demonstrated by the patient. *Do not assume the patient is taking the pills...ask!*

Look hard for adverse effects – especially those that the patient may not recognize as being drug induced. Who would ever imagine that eye drops could cause cold feet? *Ask about common adverse side effects. Consider rarer ones.*

Once you are satisfied that continuing treatment is appropriate, enter the medication on the patient's repeat file and set a review date. The review interval should be as long as is consistent with safe treatment. Most long-term medication can be reviewed annually (relying on the patient to attend for intermediate checks when these are appropriate).

The review

Reviewing medication requires some sort of consultation. It need not always be a dedicated consultation between GP and patient. It may be conducted by someone else (e.g nurse, hospital doctor). It may sometimes take place over the phone, and occasionally by post. It may be conducted opportunistically in the course of a consultation about something else. Rarely it may take place at a chance meeting in the supermarket. But it must involve some sort of communication between patient and doctor. It is impossible to conduct a real review of medication without some information about the patient's progress. Anyone who claims to have conducted a review by looking through a patient's notes that contain no new information since the last review is only deceiving himself.

The doctor should examine the whole of the patient's drug regimen and check that his records match the patient's (or carer's). If there has been a hospital admission or outpatient attendance it is also important to consider whether the drug regimen has been updated in response. Each drug should then be considered separately:

1   Is the drug effective?

2   Is the drug still needed?

3   Is the drug being taken properly?

4   Are there any adverse effects?

5   How does the patient feel about the treatment?

6   Should the drug be stopped, replaced or have the dose adjusted?

The patient should then be given a new copy of the drug list (if it has changed), and a new review date entered on the computer.

Conclusion

Repeat prescribing is a complex activity involving many people, which is almost impossible to manage perfectly. A disciplined detailed approach will improve quality of care, reduce unnecessary consultations, save resources and perhaps prevent litigation. It is worth the effort!

Further reading

Audit Commission. (1994) *A Prescription for Improvement. Towards more Rational Prescribing in General Practice.* HMSO, London.

Balint M *et al.* (1984) *Treatment or Diagnosis. A Study of Repeat Prescriptions in General Practice.* Tavistock Publications, London.

Consumers Association. Repeat Prescribing – Is it necessary and can it be safe? *Drug and Therapeutics Bulletin,* **24**(14): 54–6.

9 Formularies

Philip M Reilly

A formulary in general practice is a voluntary preferred selection of medications assembled by the practice. Several practices may be involved, and colleagues such as pharmacists and specialists, particularly pharmacologists, may also contribute.

A drug formulary may be based on the therapeutic classes as in the *BNF*. Another format consists of the selection of medications on the basis of clinical conditions. Thus the cardiovascular section would include congestive heart failure, hypertension, and so on. This format is helpful for GPs who have to contend with a wide range of conditions that may be precisely defined or be quite non-specific, such as dizziness.

Underlying assumptions

A general practice formulary is intended (Grant *et al.*, 1985):

1 to provide simple, adequate and appropriate treatment for the vast majority of patients presenting with common conditions – where the prescribing of a drug is thought necessary

2 to be useful and acceptable to a diverse group of general practitioners in a range of practice settings

3 to encourage generic prescribing where this is appropriate

4 to avoid the inclusion of any recently introduced drug until there is evidence of its superiority over standard treatment. This will not result in patients being deprived of the newest and, by implication, the best medications. The withdrawal of new preparations because of unacceptable side-effects is common enough to make general practitioners circumspect. In any case, a critical scrutiny of new preparations by the general practitioners involved in formulary construction is highly desirable for all concerned, including the patient and the pharmaceutical industry

5   to take into account the cost of drugs as an important but not paramount factor. In fact adequate treatment of, and medication for, some conditions may well increase prescribing costs. With asthma patients it may be expensive to prescribe adequate inhaled steroids, monitor the effects regularly and even make occasional appropriate referrals, but if these prevent emergency admissions, the overall cost to the NHS will be substantially reduced

6   to exclude medications that are usually initiated in hospital care (for instance, most cytotoxics). Medications for common conditions that have been recommended in hospital should be scrutinized, as the choice of preparation may not necessarily concur with the practice's formulary policy. A diplomatic, sensible and professional way of dealing with this is to ensure that the local hospital formulary contains and marks the preparations from any general practice formulary widely used locally with an asterisk. Placed prominently at the front of the hospital formulary should be a statement such as: 'Drugs marked with an asterisk (*) have been selected for inclusion in the local general practice formularies and are therefore particularly suited for general practitioner prescribing when the patient has been discharged'

7   to provide a useful tool for teaching and learning

8   to be modified predominantly by general practitioners for general practitioners on a regular basis.

Why the need for a formulary?

So large is the volume of information and so great the range of preparations used by GPs that they are in danger of being overloaded. How can prescribing – a central activity in any clinician's role – be maintained as an area of professional competence, even expertise?

Effective prescribing comprises several skills, such as being able to assimilate or access relevant pharmacological and therapeutic information, to update knowledge, as well as to cope with new concepts. Being able to communicate with patients is very important – wants and needs are not the same, and effective negotiation and education are always a part of doctor–patient relationships. Being able to maximize compliance is becoming ever more essential as chronic diseases increase in prevalence. Finally, the ability to organize and manage a repeat prescribing system operationally and clinically is vital. Repeat prescribing is a significant and perhaps permanent feature of UK general practice and can be seen, to a small extent, in most health care systems.

In dealing with many common conditions the GP is usually faced with many preparations from which to choose. Secondly, the range of choice, thanks in part to an innovative pharmaceutical industry, frequently changes. Therefore, inevitably, GPs must adopt a strategy to cope effectively as prescribers. They must become active, and develop criteria that enable them to make good selections. Such activity is rigorous, voluntary, professionally satisfying and likely to maximize good patient care – it is called **formulary construction**. Cost containment is a likely, but not inevitable, by-product; efficacy, safety and acceptability to patients should always be in evidence.

How to go about constructing a formulary

Three tasks are involved for which satisfactory answers must be found and sound policies developed.

1 Developing selection criteria for choosing medications

Each of the illnesses commonly managed by GPs will usually offer the prescriber a wide choice. At least 80% of patients in general practice with any given common illness will respond to an established medication. A small minority will require considerable therapeutic effort in effecting a cure, improvement or maintenance. Selection together with some flexibility is therefore inevitable. Provided this '80:20' rule is observed, cost containment is rarely a major issue because cost effectiveness is being addressed. The majority (about 80%) of patients receive established medications and these are likely to be cost-effective (though this does not mean that further improvement is not possible). It does not mean that they are getting cheap, second-rate medications. In dealing with the minority (20%) of patients not responding to established medications, the prescriber can be appropriately radical, outside the formulary selection. Formularies in general practice should not be inflexible.

The challenge for the prescriber is therefore to identify to which group the patient with common illness belongs – the 80% majority or the 20% minority – and to prescribe accordingly. Such a professional approach from the prescriber should also mean that patients get the medications appropriate to their clinical condition.

How, therefore, are medications selected for a practice formulary? It is relatively easy to think of characteristics a drug must possess. Being effective, safe, economic, appropriate to the condition, as well as acceptable to the patient, are all desirable characteristics. It is, however, quite a challenge to organize these features in such a way that a choice can be made between the various preparations in a given therapeutic class. A simple, though at times difficult exercise, consists in itemizing specific selection criteria, as shown in Table 9.1.

Table 9.1: Sample of specific selection criteria for different named drugs.

Specific selection criteria	Names of various medications
	Drug A Drug B Drug C Drug D etc.
Aim (in use)	
Observations	
Alternatives	
Duration of course	
Metabolism	
Interactions	
Route and dosage	
Unwanted effects	
Cost	

Selection criteria may vary in certain therapeutic classes and should be extended as much as possible so that the best choices can be made. Therapeutic classes such as non-steroidal anti-inflammatory drugs, where there are many medications, involve one sort of selection process. Choice of preparations that lower lipid levels, where there are relatively few preparations as yet, involve a different process. These processes of selection vary with almost every therapeutic class.

Many relevant prescribing issues are raised, though not all can be settled. In any case, the selection process is ongoing and is really a major learning opportunity in which doctors build up a structured approach to selection that has a wide application for established as well as new medications.

The names of medications are placed across the top of the sheet. The criteria are listed on the left hand side of the page. These criteria put pertinent questions to the selectors who may include other disciplines (for example pharmacists, pharmacologists) as well as all the practice doctors. The drugs chosen have the most acceptable profile.

The specific selection criteria may be defined as follows:

Aim: What is the aim/purpose in using the proposed medication?

Observations: What observations have to be made when using the proposed medication?

Alternatives: What are the alternatives (medication and otherwise) available?

Duration: How long does the medication have to be taken?

Metabolism: How does the body handle the medication?

Interactions: What interactions (expected and others) might be observed?

Route and dosage: Self-explanatory

Unwanted effects: What are these and how acceptable are they?

2 Getting the group (GPs and others) to work cohesively and effectively together to produce prescribing policies

When practices are observed examining their own prescribing data, they (as a group) progress or fail to progress through a series of stages:

1 defensive comments: e.g. 'we are not very good at this'

2 projective comments: e.g. 'we are the sort of practice that . . .'

3 deficiency acknowledged: this is especially seen when the group has its own data in front of it

4 dialogue: this is particularly noted when everybody knows each other's data

5 agreement/disagreement: how productive this exchange is really depends on how the practice group handles the range of committed and other views expressed

6 policy development: the practice group needs some form of working consensus and good sources of information so that members can address and complete a series of tasks

7 implementing change: such change must be carried out efficiently and in a committed manner

8 checking that change has taken place: practice organization is needed here as well as commitment.

Practice groups will not progress beyond the stage of agreement/ disagreement unless they work together regularly and in a manner that caters for the needs of the members as well as the task in hand.

It is important to ensure that as many as possible of the practice group actually do the work of setting criteria and applying them. Some of the group might later challenge the validity of the chosen criteria if, for example, an unacceptable level of compliance is found. In attempting to generate a feeling of responsibility for the criteria chosen, the practice group may enlarge and lengthen them. Such developments result in criteria that are less precise and usually less easily audited. Precise criteria are essential if data are to be used and not left unconsidered – the so-called 'orphan data'. Participants in audit respond best to specific items which, if not attained, are remedied by an education programme that is focused, personal and occurs soon after the audit exercise has stopped. Success is most likely when involvement has been active, addressing issues documented by clinical research and selected for its importance to patients' well-being and for correctability by doctor performance.

The management of change and the development of innovation are demanding. The practice group needs to know when change is really necessary. The whole process must not only seem, but actually be, possible. The impression and the reality will be more successful if the whole process is shared by all the participants. Both practice and individual practitioner identity must be reinforced.

3 Handling operational problems such as repeat prescribing

A repeat prescribing system, adequately policed, is not just acceptable but very necessary in current UK general practice. Good information systems allow repeat prescriptions to be printed by a computer with policy decisions built in, thus saving valuable time. However, the initial impact of formulary construction could be significant.

The practice will wish to consider policies as applied to patients receiving repeat prescriptions. In the light of any changes, will any or all such patients have to be seen? What explanation will be given? How can the practice ensure that such explanations will be understood? At least one third, and in some cases up to one half, of all doctor-patient contacts face to face (direct) or otherwise (indirect) are through the repeat prescribing system. The practice will have to explain change, systematically and in an acceptable way, to various categories of patients, including the elderly, the housebound, and so on. Such changes will have to be clinically indicated, as safe as possible, understood and complied with willingly, and in as informed a manner as possible.

How to maintain a practice formulary

Successful initial construction of a general practice formulary involves multidisciplinary activity as described above. Use and acceptance of the formulary is strongly related to active participation.

Such ownership can be fostered and strengthened by the formation of user groups. These groups are essentially self-directed, although they will agree to monitor a particular section of the formulary and update it as required. They can be resourced with substantial prescribing information about the particular area/therapeutic class they wish to develop. Apart from information, community pharmacists and drug information pharmacists can supply relevant data. These can be added to the detailed feedback already available through PACT in England and Wales and SPA in Scotland. Other professionals may be involved: pharmacists most commonly, but also pharmacologists.

User groups could well become a useful forum for exchange of ideas that can be collated centrally. Examples of such exchanges include:

1   the development of cost–benefit analyses that may enable the best type of choices of medication to be made

2   access to a company 'rep' or 'detail' man from the pharmaceutical industry. This may present a useful opportunity for particular companies. Occasionally, sound postmarketing surveillance studies could be carried out (see Chapter 15)

3   studies that examine issues of variation in prescribing between areas that seem similar – does such variation represent over or under treatment?

4   continuing exploration of factors (for example, age structure or specific morbidity) which may affect prescribing.

At the same time, practices participating in formulary construction will feel that they are making an effective and essential contribution to maintaining an important component of good patient care.

Conclusion

Given the range of skills required of a competent prescriber, strategies are essential. The strategy of formulary construction, implying active involvement but nevertheless voluntary in nature, represents the sort of educational, collaborative and professional activity essential for competence in prescribing. It is not a cost-containment exercise bent on giving the patient less than optimal medication.

The construction of practice formularies is not an activity inimical to the pharmaceutical industry. It represents general practitioners reclaiming fundamental areas of competence in a manner that will sustain them through their professional careers.

Further reading

Grant G B, Gregory D A and Van Zwanenberg T D. (1985) Development of a limited formulary for general practice. *Lancet,* 2: 1030–1.

Green P E. (1985) The general practice formulary – its role in rational therapeutics. *Journal of the Royal College of General Practitioners,* 35: 570–2.

Nelson A R. (1976) Orphan data and the closed loop. *New England Journal of Medicine,* 295: 617–19.

Reilly P M. (1985) *An Audit of Prescribing by Peer Review.* MD Thesis. Queen's University, Belfast.

10   The selected list scheme

Conrad M Harris

History

On April 1, 1985, a large number of medicines became unavailable for prescription by general practitioners under the NHS. The move, which had been announced in November 1984, was deeply unpopular with most doctors: some saw it as a constraint on their clinical freedom; others thought that the changes lacked any coherence and could have been improved had there been some prior consultation with the profession; and almost all believed that the real purpose of the limitation was political rather than clinical or even economic. The pharmaceutical industry was worried, and warned of the consequences both to patients and to future research and development.

The new scheme, which came into effect as Schedule 3 of the 1974 GMS Regulations, involved seven therapeutic categories:

- antacids
- laxatives
- cough and cold remedies
- analgesics for mild to moderate pain
- vitamins
- tonics
- benzodiazepines.

Within these categories, 31 preparations were deemed sufficient to meet all clinical needs, and all others were 'blacklisted'. The preparations available had to be prescribed generically, and for those that were combination drugs, co-names (e.g. coproxamol, codydramol) were invented by the Pharmacopoeial Commission to prevent prescribing by the proprietary name.

By February 1986 the 31 preparations had been increased to 129 and an Advisory Committee had been set up to advise ministers on which drugs would meet all clinical needs in the defined categories at the lowest possible cost. This included five general practitioners and representatives of hospital specialties, pharmacologists and pharmacists.

It soon became clear that there were patients with particular conditions whose clinical needs were not being met, and a special category was created to allow general practitioners to prescribe a few blacklisted drugs under specific conditions. This category later became Schedule 11 of the 1992 GMS Regulations, and currently includes five drugs. The blacklist, with many preparations, has become Schedule 10 of the same regulations (Box 10.1). Some of these preparations are considered to be foods of cosmetics – these are dealt with by the Advisory Committee on Borderline Substances.

Box 10.1: Schedule 10 drugs and Schedule 11 drugs

Schedule 10: drugs and other substances not to be prescribed for supply under pharmaceutical services

Schedule 11: drugs to be prescribed under pharmaceutical services only in specific circumstances

---

Amendments to these schedules are made from time to time by the Secretary of State, who takes advice from the Advisory Committee.

In November 1992, the Secretary of State announced the extension of the blacklisting policy – then known offiically as the Selected List Scheme – to a further ten therapeutic categories containing about 1500 preparations (Box 10.2).

She also made a significant alteration in the Advisory Committee's remit by stating that a drug would be treated as falling within one of these categories according to the purpose for which it was prescribed, even if it were not licensed for that purpose.

The extension of blacklisting into the ten new categories alarmed not only doctors and the pharmaceutical industry, but also members of the public – especially in regard to oral contraceptives and preparations used in the treating of skin conditions such as eczema: once again, therefore the response had a political dimension.

The outcome has been something of an anti-climax. More than two and a half years later, decisions have been taken in only five of the ten categories, only 63 preparations have been blacklisted, and only one of these is a

Box 10.2: The Selected List Scheme, November 1992

- anti-diarrhoeal drugs
- drugs for allergic disorders
- hypnotics and anxiolytics
- appetite suppressants
- drugs for vaginal and vulval conditions
- contraceptives
- drugs used in anaemia
- topical anti-rheumatics
- drugs acting on the ear and nose
- drugs acting on the skin.

prescription-only medicine (Ledercort cream). Forty of the 63 are proprietary topical anti-rheumatics, none of them a non-steroidal anti-inflammatory agent. Though five categories remain to be considered, the main effect of the exercise has been a number of price reductions made by pharmaceutical companies anxious to avoid the blacklisting of their products. Pharmaceutical firms complain that the way that the Advisory Committee decides upon the acceptability of such reductions is not made clear; that consideration is given only to the cost and not to the benefit of a drug; and that the Committee is not allowed to take into account the adverse impact of a company's position within the Pharmaceutical Pricing Regulation Scheme which controls its profits.

In evidence given to the House of Commons Health Committee for its report on *Priority Setting in the NHS: The NHS Drugs Budget*, published in 1994, the industry referred to its earlier warnings about the adverse effect on research and development in the therapeutic categories subjected to blacklisting, and claimed that these had been shown to be justified. An independent pharmacologist responded by noting that though only six products were added to these categories between 1986 and (April) 1994, even fewer – three – had been added in the five years before the introduction of the scheme.

The process of blacklisting

The Advisory Committee has been meeting every month to consider every licensed product in the specified categories as set out in the *British National Formulary*, together with those products that might be prescribed for the same purposes from other sections of the *Formulary*. It has to review all presentations of every preparation: oral or topical; solid or liquid; sugar-free or containing sugar; and ointments, creams and lotions. In each case it has to determine whether there is a clinical need and, if there is, which products meet that need most economically. It also has to take into consideration duration of treatment, dosage and relative efficacy.

It can take safety for granted since the preparations are licensed; relative efficacy is a matter for its judgement, which is based on submissions by the manufacturers, its own research and the specialist knowledge of its members.

For each category it draws up a list of all the preparations it will consider – a huge task, especially in the case of drugs acting on the skin. The manufacturers of each product within this list are invited to submit data and evidence for its continuing availability on NHS prescription. After considering the information supplied, the Committee makes its preliminary determinations. It informs the manufacturers about these and gives them an opportunity to make any representations they would like to have considered.

The Committee then makes decisions – sometimes after taking further evidence orally – that are notified to the manufacturers. Some lower their prices and some review the position of their products in the market; a number of products have been withdrawn.

The Committee's final recommendations are presented to the Secretary of State, who sets out a list of the intended additions to Schedule 10 in a Press Release so that members of the public have one month to comment on them. After this, the de-listed preparations are included in the Schedule, subject to parliamentary approval.

Schedule 10 and the Terms of Service

Many products included in the blacklist have been a source of hilarity – Weight Watchers' Baked Beans and communion wafers for example – but for general practitioners Schedule 10 is not a laughing matter: they can be taken before a service committee if they infringe it.

Pharmacists will often contact a doctor in time for a prescription to be amended, partly to protect the doctor and also because they do not get reimbursed for dispensing a listed preparation; several thousand banned items, however, reach the Prescription Pricing Authority every month. The PPA returns the prescriptions to the relevant FHSA, which is responsible for taking proceedings against the prescriber. It is not known how often service committees have been asked to consider such a breach of the regulations, but this is probably rare unless a prescriber has made a habit of infringing them. The FHSA's medical adviser follows up a case in the first instance.

All GPs should keep up with amendments to the Regulations that affect Schedules 10 and 11, and have them near to hand until they are sure that they know them.

The future

The Government's claim that the 1985 list saved the NHS £70 million in its first year has never been substantiated, but after ten years it is unlikely to be causing any problems. The new categories announced in 1992 were more serious in their potential effects on prescribing, though so far the outcome has been minimal. Decisions have not yet been reached about many of these categories however, and the Advisory Committee continually has to reassess those on which it has already made recommendations, because of new drugs coming on to the market and because indications for treatment may change.

The Advisory Committee seems to have been taking a conservative and uncontroversial approach to its task, and the Department of Health seems not to have been courting any professional or public outcry in this field. There are, however, still five categories for which no decisions have been announced, and plenty of scope for surprise remains. The Department of Health is considering the recommendation of the House of Commons Health Committee that blacklisting be abolished, and replaced by a whitelist containing a restricted number of preparations that may be prescribed. The response to such a controversial action could make reactions to the Selected List scheme pale into insignificance.

Meanwhile, general practitioners who want to have their concerns about the Selected List considered should write to the secretary of the Advisory Committee at Richmond House, Whitehall.

11　Controlled drugs

Jacqueline V Jolleys

Introduction

The Misuse of Drugs Act 1971 and The Misuse of Drugs Regulations 1986 define the basis of control for specific drugs (known as controlled drugs) whose misuse gives rise to social problems. The rights and responsibilities of duly registered medical practitioners are specified by these regulations. The areas of control covered by these regulations that have particular relevance to practitioners in the course of their everyday work include:

The Misuse of Drugs Act 1971

- enables and requires the Home Secretary to make regulations affecting the day to day performance of duties relating to controlled drugs by health professionals

- enables the Home Secretary to give direction prohibiting a practitioner from having in his possession, prescribing, administering, manufacturing, compounding or supplying and authorizing administration and supply of certain drugs if that practitioner:
  - has been convicted of an offence under The Misuse of Drugs Act
  - has prescribed controlled drugs in an irresponsible way
  - has contravened the Misuse of Drugs Regulations (1973) relating to notification and supply of addicts

- empowers an authorized police officer and/or practitioner (usually the Medical Adviser) to enter the premises of persons supplying controlled drugs and demand the production and inspection of books and documents relating to dealings in controlled drugs, and inspection of any stocks of controlled drugs.

The Misuse of Drugs Regulations

- enable specific classes of persons to possess, produce, supply, prescribe or administer controlled drugs in the practice of their professions

- apply controls to certain groups of drugs which are divided into five

schedules, the regulations for each schedule specifying the requirements with respect to:
- supply and possession
- storage (safe custody)
- record keeping
- prescription
- destruction

- exert requirements with respect to the importation and exportation of these selected medications in the form of licensing

- pronounce on notification of and supply to addicts.

The five schedules of controlled drugs

Schedule 1 includes:

- cannabis

- hallucinogens, e.g. lysergide, mescaline

- raw opium

- concentrate of poppy straw and coca leaf.

This schedule covers the most strictly controlled drugs. In general they have no accepted therapeutic use and practitioners have no statutory right of access to them. As such possession and supply are prohibited except in accordance with Home Office Authority, a licence from the Home Secretary is required to possess, produce, supply, offer, administer or cause to administer drugs covered by this schedule.

Schedule 2 includes:

- morphine

- diamorphine

- pethidine

- amphetamine

- cocaine

- quinalbarbitone

- glutethimide.

More than one hundred drugs are covered by this schedule, but in practical terms they are pharmaceutical opioids and amphetamines, few of which are in regular, let alone common, medical use. The use of these medications is subject to full controlled drugs requirements relating to prescriptions, safe custody, destruction, registers etc.

Schedule 3 includes

- barbiturates but not quinalbarbitone (included in schedule 2)

- mazindol

- meprobamate

- pentazocine

- phentermine

- diethylpropion

- buprenorphine.

Although subject to special prescription regulations this schedule of drugs is not subject to safe custody requirements, nor the need to keep special registers, although drug purchasers (e.g. dispensing practices) are required to retain invoices for a minimum of two years.

Schedule 4 includes:

- benzodiazepines (33 benzodiazepine tranquillizers)

- pemoline.

Schedule 4 drugs are subject to minimum control since there are no restrictions to their possession in medicinal product form. One requirement is the retention of invoices for the drugs for two years. These preparations are not subject to controlled prescription requirements nor to safe storage regulations. Temazepam is about to be moved to schedule 3.

Schedule 5 drugs

Schedule 5 exempts from most of the controls applying to schedule 2 drugs, a number of preparations that contain small quantities of some of the drugs in that schedule. Schedule 5 preparations in common use include those of codeine, hydrocodeine, morphine, medicinal opium, diphenoxylate, pholcodine, and dextropropoxyphene. Schedule 5 does not relate to any preparation designed for injection. So, whereas the injection of dihydrocodeine is covered by schedule 2, tablets containing dihydrocodeine are contained in schedule 5. Schedule 5 regulations require only that invoices are to be retained for a minimum of two years.

Commonly prescribed proprietary-named controlled drugs are listed in each edition of *The British National Formulary (BNF)*. In addition, an alphabetical list of some official preparations, as specified under The Misuse of Drugs Regulations 1985, schedules 2 and 3 are appendixed.

Supply and possession of controlled drugs

When acting in their professional capacity, several health care professional groups have authority to possess, supply and produce drugs specified in schedules 2, 3, 4 and 5. These include dentists, doctors and pharmacists. In addition, doctors and dentists may directly administer such drugs to patients. Supply of the specified classes of controlled drugs is restricted to those who may lawfully possess them, including patients to whom they are correctly and properly prescribed. With respect to administration of controlled drugs that have been prescribed in general practice, a registered general nurse who is a sister or acting sister in charge of a nursing home or a general practitioner ward, may supply a controlled drug for administration to a patient in that nursing home or ward. Similarly a registered general nurse or district nursing sister may administer a controlled drug to a patient in accordance with the direction of the practitioner. A community midwife is permitted under The Misuse of Drugs Regulations to possess and administer any controlled drug for the purpose of pursuing her profession; in practice this limits possession to two drugs, pethidine and pentazocine.

A patient may possess a drug in schedule 2 or 3 for his own use. It must have been correctly prescribed for him by a practitioner, and once supplied becomes the property of the patient. A person other than the patient for whom the drug is prescribed may possess the controlled drug if he/she is conveying it to the patient for whom it is prescribed. A patient or his representative is also authorized under the regulations to convey any unwanted supply of the controlled drug to a practitioner or pharmacist for the purpose of destruction, although the drug remains the property of the patient for whom it was prescribed and the practitioner or pharmacist becomes the patient's representative. As such the returned, unwanted medication should not be entered in the practitioner's or pharmacist's controlled drugs registers but should merely be stored safely while awaiting destruction.

When a patient who has been prescribed controlled drug medication dies, the unwanted supplies of controlled drug legally become the property of the executors who must arrange for their destruction.

A doctor must not supply, administer or authorize the administration of cocaine, heroin, dipipanone or any salts to someone whom he considers addicted to the drug, or has reasonable grounds to suspect is so addicted, except for the treatment of injury or organic disease or under licence from the Home Secretary. A GP may administer or supply these drugs to addicts if the supply or administration is authorized by another doctor under and in accordance with a licence issued to him by the Home Secretary (see Prescribing for addicts, page 109).

Requisition of controlled drugs

Before schedule 2 or 3 drugs can be supplied to a medical practitioner, e.g. for emergency use in the surgery or in his emergency bag, a requisition is required. To satisfy the regulations the requisition must:

- be signed by the recipient (practitioner)
- state the purpose for which the drug is being supplied
- state the name, address and profession of the recipient
- state the quantity to be supplied (not required to be both in words and figures).

Prior to supplying the controlled drug, the supplier is required to satisfy himself that the requisition is genuine and that the recipient is engaged in the profession stated. If the practitioner has sent someone to collect the supplies of the controlled drug on his behalf, there must also be a signed statement empowering the person to take receipt of the drugs. Once again the supplier is charged with the responsibility of ensuring that the statement is genuine.

In an emergency a practitioner can obtain supplies of a controlled drug without immediately supplying a signed requisition; however the practitioner must undertake to deliver the signed requisition within 24 hours of receiving the drug. Failure to do so constitutes an offence under the Misuse of Drugs Regulations.

Storage (safe custody) of controlled drugs

The Misuse of Drugs (Safe Custody) Regulations (1973) requires all controlled drugs, other than those specified, to be kept in a locked receptacle. This regulation in fact specifically covers controlled drugs in schedule 2 but not schedule 3 (with the exception of buprenorphine and diethylpropion), or schedules 4 and 5.

In terms of the law, the regulations require the specified controlled drugs to be kept in a locked receptacle (e.g. doctor's drug case) which can be opened only by the practitioner or someone authorized by him to open it. The courts have ruled that for the purposes of the regulations, having the controlled drugs in a bag in a locked car or locked car boot is not sufficient, and that to follow the regulations controlled drugs must be kept in a locked bag in a locked car.

It has further been recommended that the bag is stored out of view of the public (i.e. in the car boot). If the controlled drugs are carried in an estate car it is suggested that the locked bag is not left in the unoccupied car, or that a car safe in which the bag is locked is bolted to the car subframe. Police with responsibility for controlled drugs commend the fitting of car safes in saloon cars for additional security. Furthermore they request doctors not to advertise the fact that the car belongs to a doctor since this may encourage drug-related car crime.

It is recommended that controlled drugs storage is kept to a minimum at surgery premises. In surgeries and, in particular, dispensing practices where a supply of controlled drugs is necessary, these must be kept in a locked cabinet, sited away from the public. It is recommended that a locked controlled drugs cabinet is secured to the wall of a room, where access is restricted to surgery staff, and which can be locked when unoccupied. Special drugs cabinets are available for purchase.

Record keeping

Up-to-date records of controlled drugs must be maintained, both for those kept on the premises and those relating to the doctor's emergency bag, in accordance with the Misuse of Drugs Regulations.

Schedule 1 and 2 drugs

All transactions with respect to drugs specified under schedules 1 and 2 have to be recorded. This does not apply to the prescribing of schedule 1 and 2 drugs where the prescription is dispensed by a pharmacist and the practitioner never sees or handles the medication, since the drug is initially the property of the pharmacist and then that of the patient.

To satisfy requirements as laid down in the regulations the register must:

- be bound (not loose leaf). Any bound book will do so long as it is appropriately ruled and the columns are properly headed. It need not be printed

- be used solely for the purposes of controlled drug transactions

- be preserved for two years from the date of the last transaction

- use separate parts of the register for each class of drug with separate pages for each type of preparation and each strength

- have the class of drug to which any page relates given at the head of each page

- be set out in conformity with schedule 6 to the Misuse of Drugs Regulations 1985, with separation of entries governing obtaining drugs and supplying the same

- be a record of drugs kept at the one set of premises completed by all the doctors working as a group. Alternatively each partner may keep individual controlled drugs registers, but both joint and individual records should not be kept concurrently.

Note: If drugs are kept at more than one surgery a separate register must be kept for each site. Furthermore a practitioner must have a separate register to cover controlled drugs in his emergency bag, that must be kept with the bag. Registers that comply with requirements can be purchased from the National Pharmaceutical Association and Jordans of Liverpool (Figure 11.1).

In practice many practitioners prefer to record more information than is required. Batch numbers and a total stock balance are helpful in tracing individual stock items, but are not mandatory. Having a page-numbered, indexed register facilitates finding the appropriate section. The author de-

Part I
Entries to be made in case of obtaining

	NAME ADDRESS			
Date on which supply received	Of person or firm from whom obtained		Amount obtained	Form in which obtained

Part II
Entries to be made in case of supply

	NAME ADDRESS	Particulars as to licence or authority of person or firm supplied to be in possession		Form in which
Date on which the transaction was effected	Of person or firm supplied		Amount supplied	supplied

Figure 11.1 An example of a controlled drugs register as shown in the *Department of Health Guide to the Misuse of Drugs Act 1971* and the *Misuse of Drugs Regulations*.

signed her own register which more than covered requirements, with a separate double sheet for each scheduled preparation, and also gave a running stock total and columns to allow recording of drug destruction (see Figure 11.2).

According to the regulations entries must be made:

- in chronological order

- must not be cancelled, altered or obliterated

- corrections must be made by a marginal note or footnote giving the date of the correction

- written in indelible ink

- be made on the date of the transaction, or if not practical the next day.

The regulations do not require entries to be made for controlled drugs returned to a doctor or a pharmacist for the purpose of destruction.

Drug name

Proprietary

Pharmacological

| Date | Stock in | | | | | Stock out | | | | Signed | Witness | Total stock/ balance |
	Amount	Batch no.	Expiry date	Source/supplier (name/address)		Amount	Batch no.	Expiry date	Supplied to (name/ address) disposal			

Figure 11.2 Register for recording drug information.

Schedule 3 drugs

Invoices and other records must be kept for transactions relating to those drugs, specifying the quantity of drug obtained and supplied, unless the supply was made under NHS prescription. In effect this requirement rarely affects practices other than dispensing practices.

The regulations require information to be kept relating to:

- date of transaction

- person by whom or to whom the drug was supplied.

In practice retention of the invoices and copies of private prescriptions and requisitions retained for a period of a least two years suffices.

Inspection of records and drug stocks by an authorized person

The Secretary of State for Health may require or authorize in writing another person (FHSA Medical Adviser) to require the practitioner on occasion to produce registers, documentation and stocks relating to controlled drugs in his/her possession. Furthermore, the Home Secretary authorizes Inspectors of the Home Office Drugs Branch and a number of others who may also demand these details. Failure to comply or to produce appropriate records constitutes an offence.

Prescription

The regulations cover prescriptions for schedule 2 and 3 drugs. The regulations aim to minimize the forgery or alteration of prescriptions. When writing an FP10 for such drugs covered by The Misuse of Drugs Regulations a number of principal legal requirements apply. The prescription must:

- be written in indelible ink
- be legible
- be signed by the prescriber with his/her usual signature
- be dated by the prescriber (a computer-generated date is not acceptable although a rubber-stamped date or typewritten date by the prescriber is acceptable)

- include the patient's name and address, preferably handwritten, although this need not be so

- include in the prescriber's handwriting

  – the name, strength, form (i.e. tabs or caps) and dose of the preparation
  – dose to be taken
  – the total quantity to be dispensed, in both figures and words.

If the prescription is to be dispensed in instalments, in the prescriber's own handwriting, the prescription must specify the number of instalments, the interval between the same, and the instalment quantities. In all cases the total quantity or number of dosage units must be handwritten in words and figures (see Figure 11.3). Prescriptions ordering 'repeats' are not permitted.

There is a notable exception to the schedule 2 and 3 drugs with respect to prescription regulations, and that relates to the prescribing of phenobarbitone or phenobarbitone-containing preparations. With respect to the prescribing of phenobarbitone alone the requirement to handwrite the prescription is waivered and a computer-generated prescription is acceptable so long as it is separately dated by the signatory.

It should be noted that it is an offence to issue a prescription that does not comply with the requirements of the regulations and a pharmacist is not allowed to dispense the prescription for a controlled drug unless all the information required by law is given on the prescription.

Prescription form FP10 (MDA)

As the number of drug addicts rises, more are being treated in the community by specially licenced general practitioners (see Prescribing for addicts, page 109). In order to prescribe small amounts of medication on a daily basis the correct use of prescription form FP10 (MDA) is encouraged. This is the appropriate form for prescribing drugs for addicts. The form FP10 (MDA) is similar to an ordinary FP10. It can be ordered specially from the FHSA. Those issued to general practitioners are pale blue whereas those for hospital use are pink. Where it differs from the ordinary FP10 is that it has an additional sheet on which the pharmacist records the actual dispensing of the drug.

Prescribing on an FP10 (MDA)

- The prescription must be written in accordance with the Misuse of Drugs Regulations as for any controlled drug.

- The prescriber must state the number of instalments for the supply of the drug and the interval in between, taking into account closing of the pharmacy. (It may be easier to specify the actual dates of dispensing.).

- The total quantity of drug ordered must not exceed that required for fourteen days' supply.

- No other drugs or preparations may be prescribed on FP10 (MDA).

Dispensing an FP10 (MDA)

Dispensing an FP10 (MDA) is specialized and requires the pharmacist to:

- dispense the prescription in accordance with the intervals and quantities specified by the prescriber

- record each supply in the controlled drugs register

- submit the prescription to the Prescription Pricing Authority at the end of the month

- record the date of supply, the item and the quantity dispensed on the FP10 (MDA) and to initial each record.

Both a dispensing and a controlled drug fee are payable for each instalment dispensed.

Prescribing for addicts

In order to prescribe diamorphine (heroin), cocaine and dipipanone (Diconal) for addicts, the Misuse of Drugs (Notification of and Supply to Addicts) Regulations 1973 requires the medical practitioner to hold a special licence, issued by the Home Secretary. All other practitioners must refer their addicts to a treatment centre.

Good practice requires, whenever possible, for the addict to:

- select a conveniently-sited pharmacy

- be introduced personally by a staff member from the treatment centre to the pharmacist (who has agreed to supply the addict)

- collect supplies on a daily basis as prescribed by the doctor who sends

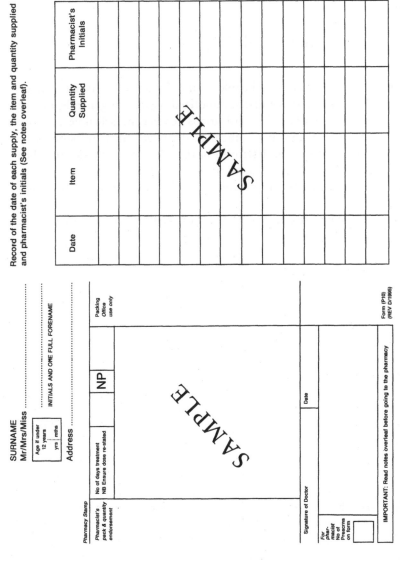

Record of the date of each supply, the item and quantity supplied and pharmacist's initials (See notes overleaf).

Date	Item	Quantity Supplied	Pharmacist's Initials

SURNAME
Mr/Mrs/Miss ....

INITIALS AND ONE FULL FORENAME

Age if under 12 years
yrs | mths

Address ....

Pharmacy Stamp

Pharmacist's pack & quantity endorsement

No of days treatment
NB Ensure dose re-stated

NP

Packing Office use only

SAMPLE

Signature of Doctor   Date

For pharmacist
No of Prescrns on form

IMPORTANT: Read notes overleaf before going to the pharmacy

Form (P10)
(REV D/1990)

Figure 11.3 Sample of (Form FP10 (MDA)) must be ordered specially from the FHSA. Those issued by the hospital are pink and those used in general practice are pale blue.

prescriptions [FP10 (MDA)] for weekly (or two-weekly) supplies to the pharmacy by post.

Destruction of controlled drugs

According to the regulations schedule 1 and 2 controlled drugs can be destroyed only in the presence of an authorized person. In general practice this means that any out-of-date medications covered by schedule 2, stock surplus to requirement and any controlled drugs returned by patients or patients' relatives, have to be destroyed in the presence of the local police drugs officer or the authorized medical adviser. It may be wise to treat schedule 3 drugs similarly or dispose through local returned medicines schemes.

For schedule 2 controlled drugs, a record of the destruction must be kept specifying:

- name of drug destroyed
- strength of the drug
- date of destruction
- quantity destroyed.

Where the drug is out-of-date stock and is recorded in the controlled drugs register, the remaining balance of in-date stock has to be counted and signed for. The record is signed by the doctor and the authorized person.

Under the Misuse of Drugs Regulations, once prescribed, the controlled drugs become the property of the patient. Patients may destroy any control-led drugs left over in their possession once medical treatment has ceased. If the quantity is large, or if they so wish, they may have the destruction supervised by an authorized person. Where the patient or patient's relative has returned the drugs to a pharmacist or a doctor, once again it should be emphasized that there is no legal requirement to make a record of their destruction under the Misuse of Drugs Regulations. Often professionals prefer a record of the destruction to be made, with the destruction witnessed by an authorized person, in order that proof exists of the fate of the drugs.

Notification of addicts

The Misuse of Drugs (Notification of and Supply to Addicts) Regulations 1973 require any doctor in England, Scotland and Wales who attends a person whom the doctor considers or has reasonable grounds to suspect is addicted to any of 14 notifiable drugs, within seven days of the attendance, to furnish in writing particulars of that person to:

The Chief Medical Officer
Home Office, Drugs Branch
Queen Anne's Gate
London SW1H 9AT

In Northern Ireland notification is made to:

The Chief Medical Officer
Department of Health and Social Services
Dundonald House
Belfast
BT4 3SF

Notification is not required if a practitioner believes in good faith that the administration of the drug or drugs concerned is necessary for the purpose of treating organic disease or injury.

The regulations stipulate that a person is to be regarded as an addict if he has, as a result of repeated administration, become so dependent on the drug that he has 'the overpowering desire for the administration of it to be continued'.

Notification is required in respect of the following preparations:

cocaine   dextromoramide
diamorphine   dipipanone (contained in Diconal tablets)
hydrocodone   hydromorphone
levanorphanol   methadone
morphine   opium
oxycodone   pethidine
phenazocine   piritramide.

When notifying the Chief Medical Officer the following particulars of the patient are required:

● name and address

- sex

- date of birth

- NHS number (if known)

- date of attendance

- names of drug(s) of addiction

- whether patient injects any drugs (relates to all drugs, not just notifiable ones).

All information notifying of addicts, supplied by doctors, is treated as confidential and the information is collated in an Index of Addicts, which is maintained in the Home Office. It is good medical practice to check all new cases of addiction, or suspected addiction, with the Index, before prescribing or supplying controlled drugs, since this safeguards against addicts getting supplies simultaneously from two different sources. Information contained in the Index of Addicts is available to GPs on a confidential basis by telephoning 0171 273 2213. The doctor will be asked to identify himself and information will be telephoned back to the doctor who made the enquiry, by lay staff, who are not qualified to give advice on the clinical management of cases.

For as long as the practitioner continues to attend and treat an addict, notification of that addict should continue to be submitted at 12 monthly intervals.

Further reading

Advisory Council on the Misuse of Drugs. (1983) *Security of Controlled Drugs.* HMSO, London.
Dale J R and Appelbie G E. (1983) *Pharmacy Law and Ethics* (3rd edn). The Pharmaceutical Press, London.
Lord R. (1984) *Controlled drugs – law and practice.* Consulting editor; Christopher Sumner, Butterworth, London.
Wells F O (ed), D'Arcy P F and Harron D W G (exec. eds). (1992) *Medicines: Responsible Prescribing.* Queens University, Belfast.

12 Prescribing advisers and budgets

David J D Sleator

Introduction

The quality and cost of prescribing in general practice have been given considerable emphasis in the recent changes within the NHS and all FHSAs/ Health Commissioning Agencies (HCs) are expected to have access to professional advice on prescribing matters. There are also professionally qualified advisers on prescribing at both the NHS Executive and at Regional Health Authorities/Regional Offices (RHAs/ROs). At most FHSAs/HCs prescribing advisers are responsible for setting, or recommending, prescribing budgets for practices. However, decisions in other parts of the NHS may influence the allocation of budgets considerably, and to understand the role of professional advisers in setting budgets at practice level, it is necessary to consider some of these factors, and the effects they may have.

Background

Prescribing cost targets were introduced for all practices on 1 April 1991. They had been announced in the White Paper 'Working for Patients', and detailed further in 'Improving Prescribing'.

Successful introduction of these targets for prescribing costs was dependent on a number of other factors, in particular the earlier development of PACT (Prescribing Analysis and Cost) reports which were first introduced in 1988. While a system of providing some feedback to GPs on their prescribing costs already existed, the introduction of PACT meant that all GPs began to receive regular reports on their prescribing, and very detailed information could be obtained with ease.

By the time budgetary targets were being set and introduced, practices had become used to receiving these reports, and GPs had appropriate information available to enable them to analyse their own prescribing in detail, and to discuss the question of budget allocations with the FPC (now FHSA) from a firm knowledge base.

PACT data were also made available to FPCs, which were given responsibility for encouraging GPs to give increased emphasis to prescribing issues. This led to the appointment of professionally-qualified prescribing advisers to FPCs, from 1990 onwards. Initially most FPCs appointed medical advisers, but increasingly pharmacists have also been involved. The numbers and mix of these professional staff varies from FHSA to FHSA, as does the range of their responsibilities, but most FHSAs now have both medical and pharmaceutical advisers involved in prescribing issues and budget setting.

The Role of the NHS Executive

Planned national prescribing expenditure is determined centrally and allocations are made to RHAs/ROs by the NHS Executive. The total allocated to each RHA/RO has a direct effect on the amount available to local FHSAs, as the total of the budgets allocated to each of the FHSAs in a region is expected normally not to exceed the overall figure allocated to the RHA/RO.

In addition to the total budget allocation, policy changes by the NHS Executive may also directly affect the setting and level of practice budgets. For example, since April 1995 a number of 'care packages' can no longer be prescribed by GPs, and therefore a number of practices with patients requiring such therapies had an equivalent reduction in their budgets as a direct consequence.

Each year the NHS Executive also issues guidance on the setting of budgets which affects the actions of both RHA/ROs and FHSAs. The guidance may range from broad objectives to be addressed to fairly detailed requirements on specific prescribing targets. Examples have ranged from encouragement to develop incentive schemes for non-fundholding practices, to detailed advice about the contents of the corporate contract between each FHSA and its RHA/RO, which identifies the areas to be prioritized by the FHSA with its practices.

The role of RHAs/ROs

RHA/ROs vary in their approach to the distribution of the budgets provided to them by the NHS Executive, some providing allocations to FHSAs based directly on the guidance provided by the NHS Executive, while others adjust allocations based on their knowledge of local circumstances. Both approaches have their merits.

Treating each FHSA in the same way has the benefit of being 'even handed', and omits subjective evaluation of the performance of each FHSA and its practices. This approach perhaps recognizes the fact that there is a great deal about the variation in prescribing patterns between FHSAs that is still not understood. Alternatively, allocating budgets to each FHSA on an individual basis, within the overall RHA/RO figure, has the major advantage of allowing for any local changes that may affect prescribing costs.

Another important role of the RHA/RO has been to hold a contingency prescribing fund for fundholding practices. While the way in which budgets are set is the same for fundholding and non-fundholding practices, the prescribing allocation to fundholders is 'real' in that it forms part of the total practice fund. The contingency reserve held at RHA/RO level has been seen as a pool of money to meet exceptional prescribing costs for which an individual practice could not reasonably plan: for example an increase in list size, or a patient starting on a particularly expensive therapy. Prescribing advisers at the RHA/RO help set the criteria for bids for contingency reserve funds, and decide the amount of any allocation. This is an important aspect of managing exceptional prescribing costs, but no change is made to the budget allocation during the year, and so performance against budget is monitored in exactly the same way as for non-fundholders. Contingency reserves for non-fundholding practices were first made available in 1994–5, and it is probable that these will be held at FHSA/HC level for both fundholding and non-fundholding practices in future.

The RHA/RO is also responsible for monitoring performance at FHSA/HC level. RHA/RO officers are in regular contact with FHSAs/HCs, and reviews of progress against budget allocations, and of other prescribing issues, particularly the corporate contract, are undertaken. The ongoing changes in the NHS suggest that this monitoring role is likely to increase.

The role of FHSAs/HCs

Professional advisers at FHSAs/HCs

While the backgrounds of professional advisers at FHSAs vary considerably, all advisers are provided with both training and information to help them in their prescribing role.

The Medical Advisers Support Centre (MASC) co-ordinates, and provides, much of the training available to both medical and pharmaceutical advisers. Most advisers use the training organized by MASC, and so have been able to develop contacts with professional colleagues.

The Medicines Resource Centre (MeReC), the Prescribing Research Unit, and the Management Services Information Systems (MSIS) Development Unit all provide support to these training activities, and each also works directly with FHSA advisers. MeReC, in particular, is well known to GPs, who receive regular prescribing bulletins from them.

Practice visits

Visiting practices to discuss prescribing is a large element of the work of most FHSA/HC prescribing advisers. While there are many other prescribing activities in which they may become involved, for example attending hospital drug and therapeutic committees, or helping develop joint formularies, practice visits continue to be of great importance. The majority of visits will cover not only issues specific to the practice, but also other general prescribing matters and local priorities. Before the visit, analysis of the practice's own prescribing patterns will be undertaken, and areas for discussion identified. A considerable amount of information is available to advisers to help them in this task.

In addition to the standard PACT reports available to practices, FHSAs have access to an electronic system provided by the Prescription Pricing Authority (PPA) called PACTLINE, which provides information, at BNF therapeutic section level, on a monthly basis. A newer system, named FEPACT, has recently been introduced that enables prescribing information, as detailed as a specific drug formulation, to be obtained on individual practices. The ability to examine the trends and patterns of prescribing with these systems is becoming increasingly important.

The visit should be seen by both the practice and the FHSA/HC adviser as an opportunity to exchange information and ideas. It is an excellent opportunity for the practice to advise the FHSA/HC of local circumstances.

Setting a practice budget

Good information is central to setting equitable practice budgets, but both general, or policy, issues and local factors need to be considered. The total budget allocated to the FHSA is an important determining factor for the general level of practice budgets, as the total of the budgets set for all the practices is not expected to normally exceed the overall FHSA allocation.

It is very important to reflect the individual characteristics and circumstances of the practice when setting the budget. Information about the practice may be obtained from a variety of sources, including that already held by the FHSA, for example, from patient registration. Prescribing information from the PPA, and information provided by the practice itself, are of particular importance.

Most professional advisers at FHSAs/HCs see their role as promoting high quality prescribing and helping to reduce unnecessary prescribing costs; they will adjust individual practice budgets on a range of factors, and not merely use an average uplift for all practices. While the starting point for budget setting will be the historic costs of the practice, advisers will also look at the prescribing pattern and make judgements, based on their knowledge of each practice, about where potential savings, or increased costs, may be expected. In this way the quality and cost effectiveness of the prescribing of each practice can be reflected in the budget set. While many factors may influence a change in the prescribing cost in a practice, the actual cost which a practice has incurred reflects all the current factors including, of course, the variation between doctors that always occurs.

Relevant information about a local practice may come to the attention of the FHSA professional advisers, but each practice should ensure that it has informed the FHSA of major changes which have occurred, or are expected, within the practice. Some of the more important areas are considered below.

Practice list size

Practice list size is, not surprisingly, of fundamental importance when considering practice prescribing costs. Changes in total list size are not usually very rapid, but even a small percentage change can be expected to alter prescribing costs. Although prescribing costs per patient, or prescribing unit, are available from PACT, and PACTLINE, each practice should ensure that FHSA/HC professional advisers are aware of significant changes, as the information made available to the PPA by FHSAs may not always be as up to date as that of the practice. Changes late in the financial year, or expected changes associated, for example, with new housing developments, are unlikely to be allowed for in the budget unless the FHSA/HC is informed.

Practice demography

Apart from the number of patients in a practice, the one variable which is known to have a major influence on prescribing costs within practices is the age/sex distribution of the practice population. It is well recognized that, on average, elderly patients receive more prescriptions than younger patients.

The most frequently used baseline figure to judge practices' prescribing costs is the net ingredient cost (NIC) per prescribing unit (each patient under $65 = 1$ unit, each patient 65 and over $= 3$ units). This is the factor used to provide the comparative data included in PACT reports. However most would agree that the prescribing unit is no longer suitable for current needs. The ASTRO-PU (age, sex and temporary resident originated prescribing unit) was developed to help allow total costs to be assessed in a way which was more sensitive to the different population characteristics of individual practices. Other work, based on prescribing patterns by age and sex in individual therapeutic groups, has also been undertaken and further developments can be expected (see Chapter 4). These can all be used to help assess the quality and cost of prescribing in a practice. Each practice will know the characteristics of its patient population, and an understanding of the effects this is likely to have on prescribing patterns not only presents an opportunity for evaluation and audit of prescribing within the practice, but can be used to support any request for additional budgetary allocations.

Quality initiatives

National or local initiatives are likely to alter prescribing costs, either up or down, and this should be recognized in setting budgets. One quality area, in particular, which has been looked at within many FHSAs/HCs, has been prescribing for asthma. Most professional advisers would accept that practices developing more preventive care for asthma patients are likely to have an increase in costs, and many have specifically allowed for this when setting budgets. Therefore, practices planning specific programmes designed to bring about improvements in patient care, and that have prescribing cost implications, should bring these to the attention of the FHSA/HC so that they can be reflected in the budget.

Expensive drugs

In recent years there has been a considerable increase in the number of products being prescribed by GPs that in the past would probably have been prescribed by hospital units. Some of these products can be extremely expensive, and will certainly need to be taken into account to achieve a fair prescribing budget. Each practice should keep a list of such drugs and ensure that it is considered by the FHSA/HC.

Other new commitments

There are some situations where changes to the practice population may occur that will have a major influence on prescribing cost, but that would not necessarily be obvious from routinely available information. Examples include practices that begin to look after elderly patients in a nursing or residential home, or that take on a group of patients with special medical needs. While little information exists yet to enable very precise allowances to be made for such groups of patients, reasonable adjustments should be achievable.

The expected role of commissioning agencies

Prescribing is one aspect of a much wider picture of care provision within the NHS. The expected cost of prescribing in general practice is determined centrally each year, and there seems little doubt that any 'excessive' prescribing will result in less funds being available for other parts of the NHS. Joint DHA/FHSA Health Commissioning Agencies should enable service provision to be considered as a whole. Indeed, the possibility that developments may not occur because prescribing costs have exceeded targets will mean that prescribing is a high priority for Health Commissioning Agencies, and should ensure that some of the prescribing difficulties that arise at the primary/secondary care interface are tackled.

Guidance from the Department of Health in 1994 indicated that health authorities should ensure that hospital-led prescribing is appropriate in relation to general practice, and stressed the importance of the issues surrounding the introduction of new therapeutic products. Both these are areas where the Commissioning Agencies' policies could have a considerable effect on practice prescribing costs, and hence budgets.

The appropriateness of hospital-led prescribing

To respond to this, Health Commissioning Agencies will probably further develop the prescribing aspects of their contracts with provider units. Such contracts should be able to remove, or at least minimize, some of the prescribing problems that have arisen recently between primary and secondary care. Areas which could be tackled by this approach might include:

- the provision of prescriptions to patients being discharged from hospital or attending out-patient departments

- drugs bought cheaply by hospitals that are very much more expensive in the community

- reducing the wastage involved in the destruction of drugs brought into hospital by patients

- joint prescribing and management guidelines between primary and secondary care

- clinical responsibility for prescribing drugs that need sophisticated monitoring and specialist input.

The introduction of new drugs

Health Commissioning Agencies are likely to take an increasing role in deciding what services, including prescribing, they wish to purchase on behalf of their populations. There have been a number of valuable therapeutic advances in recent years. Sometimes a completely new type of therapy becomes available before it is clear which patients will benefit from its use, and it may also be very expensive. In these circumstances Commissioning Agencies are likely to want to work with clinicians to evaluate the likely benefits for patients, and reach agreement on the introduction of the product and audit of its use. A wide range of professionals, including prescribing advisers, is likely to be involved in these discussions.

Conclusion

The availability of high-quality information is central to the setting of a fair and equitable budget for each practice. Setting prescribing budgets at practice level is a mixture of a 'bottom-up' process (i.e. the identified or perceived needs of a practice population) and a 'top-down' process (i.e. overall planned prescribing expenditure within the NHS, and other policy issues). All these factors may have an effect on primary care prescribing costs and need to be taken into account by professional advisers when setting practice budgets.

Further reading

Crompton B. (1995) GPs need more PUs for nursing home patients. *Prescriber*, 6(1): 44–5.

Crump B J, Panton R, Drummond M F, Marchment M and Hawkes R A. (1995) Transferring the costs of expensive treatments from secondary to primary care. *BMJ*, **310**: 509–12.

Department of Health. (1990) *Improving Prescribing*. Department of Health, London.

Naish J, Sturdy P and Toon P. (1995) Appropriate prescribing in asthma and its related cost in east London. *BMJ*, **310**: 97–100.

Panton R. (1993) FHSAs and Prescribing. *BMJ*, **306**: 310–14.

Roberts S and Harris C M. (1993) Age, sex, and temporary resident originated prescribing units (ASTRO-PUs): new weightings for analysing prescribing of general practices in England. *BMJ*, **307**: 485–8.

Secretaries of State for Health, Wales, Northern Ireland and Scotland. (1989) *Working for Patients. Indicative Prescribing Budgets for General Medical Practitioners*. HMSO, London.

Sleator D J D. (1993) Towards accurate prescribing analysis in general practice: accounting for the effects of practice demography. *Br J Gen Pract*, **43**: 102–6.

13 Dispensing in general practice

David E Pickersgill

The term 'dispensing doctor' may well conjure up an image of the ruddy-faced, tweed-clad, rustic GP, standing outside some isolated cottage counting tablets out from the back of his Land Rover. Whilst this scenario may occur in some instances, dispensing in general practice has to be just as sophisticated and modern as dispensing in a high street pharmacy. It is worth remembering also that every general practitioner is required by the NHS Pharmaceutical Services Regulations to dispense medicines to their patients in certain circumstances. In the space of one short chapter it will not be possible to consider in depth all the aspects of running a dispensing practice, but the following paragraphs will touch on the major matters that need to be borne in mind and should stimulate those with a real interest in dispensing to read one of the more substantive volumes on this subject.

The regulations

Regulation 19 of the Pharmaceutical Services Regulations 1992 (SI 1992 No. 662) requires GPs to provide drugs that are needed for the immediate treatment of a patient before the patient can otherwise obtain a supply and also permits doctors to supply appliances or drugs to patients that they personally administer.

Provision of pharmaceutical services for immediate treatment or personal administration

19 A doctor –
   (a) shall provide to a patient any appliance or drug, not being a Scheduled drug, where such provision is needed for the immediate treatment of that patient before a provision can otherwise be obtained; and
   (b) may provide to a patient any appliance or drug, not being a Scheduled drug, which he personally administers or applies to that patient.

However most people understand 'dispensing doctor' to mean those doctors who supply all the drugs and appliances that their patients may need, providing that the patients are on their dispensing list. This is covered in

Regulation 20 of the Pharmaceutical Regulations (SI 1992 No. 662) under the arrangements for the provision of pharmaceutical services by doctors.

Arrangements for provision of pharmaceutical services by doctors

20–(1) Where a patient–

(a) satisfies an FHSA that he would have serious difficulty in obtaining any necessary drugs or appliances from a pharmacy by reason of distance or inadequacy of means of communication; or

(b) is resident in a controlled locality*, at a distance of more than one mile from any pharmacy, and one of the conditions specified in paragraph (2) is satisfied in his case,

he may at any time request in writing the doctor on whose list he is included to provide him with pharmaceutical services.

Obtaining permission to dispense

The subject of dispensing by doctors has long been a bone of contention between the medical and pharmaceutical professions. After many years of heated debate the matter was ultimately considered by Sir Cecil Clothier QC, (who subsequently became the Parliamentary Ombudsman for Health), and the current regulations governing who can dispense and when, are based on the recommendations that he made. Essentially, the area in which a doctor wishes to dispense has to be classified as rural in nature and, having been so classified, any patients who wish to obtain their medicines from their doctor must apply to do so in writing and must live at least one mile from the nearest pharmacy. Any doctor who is considering an application to start dispensing would be well advised to consult his Local Medical Committee (LMC) secretary long before putting pen to paper and to read carefully the written guidance which the General Medical Services Committee of the BMA (GMSC) has produced to help doctors in preparing their applications. The regulations are extremely complex and almost always such applications are opposed by local pharmacists.

The dispensary

Assuming that consent to dispense has been granted, consideration must be

---

*A controlled locality is defined as an area which the FHSA or the Appeal Unit has determined is rural in character in accordance with the Pharmaceutical Services Regulations 1992.

given to providing a suitable room within the surgery premises to serve as a dispensary. It goes without saying that it should be conveniently located as near as possible to the entrance to the surgery premises, so that patients calling to collect medicines do not need to cross crowded waiting rooms or proceed further into the surgery premises. Adequate stout shelving is required for the storage of most tablets and medicines, and there are a number of purpose-built pharmacy shelving units that can be purchased from major shop fitters. Cupboard and drawer space will be required for the storage of bulk items, catheters, dressings, external appliances, etc., and secure locked storage will be required for controlled drugs. Although most tablets and medicines may be stored at room temperature, some drugs do require storage in a refrigerator and space should be provided for this facility. A sink and lots of bench top space are essential. There are numerous electronic machines available for counting tablets that are dispensed from bulk containers, although increasingly tablets are now supplied in blister calendar packs. Likewise, most medicines are supplied in standard patient pack sizes and do not need decanting from larger containers, although some medicines, particularly antibiotics, are supplied as dry powder and need precise amounts of water measuring out to mix them up.

There are a number of labelling machines available and many general practice computer systems will now enable the doctor's desk top terminal to be linked to a terminal in the dispensary, so that at the same time as a prescription is being printed in the consulting room, a label will be produced in the dispensary.

Dispensary staff

Whilst in many practices the doctors themselves will undertake a large proportion of the dispensing, most group practices in rural areas will wish to employ at least one dispenser. Staff with dispensing experience can often be recruited from community or hospital pharmacies, and they may already possess a nationally-recognized qualification as a pharmacy technician. However, there are a number of courses organized for doctors' dispensers, many organized locally by FHSAs or pharmaceutical companies, and there is also a very good distance learning course organized through the Dispensing Doctors' Association and the People's College. It is important that dispensing staff understand their responsibilities in relation to supplying drugs to patients and also have an understanding about the ordering and storage of drugs, how to deal with prescriptions and send them to the PPA, and the regulations in relation to the storage and dispensing of controlled drugs. In this respect it is, perhaps, worth making mention of the need to have a controlled drugs register in which details are kept of all controlled drugs that are received into the practice and also of the drugs that are dispensed or taken out in the doctors' bags. A suitable register is obtainable from the Royal Pharmaceutical Society of Great Britain (see Chapter 11).

Obtaining supplies

Most dispensing doctors will deal with one principal wholesaler. Most wholesalers will offer some form of discount scheme, often charging doctors the full rate for the first thousand pounds worth of drugs purchased in any particular month, with discounts then being worked out on a sliding scale, depending on the total value of the order. In recent years many pharmaceutical companies have become more willing to deal direct with dispensing doctors and this enables doctors to take advantage of the attractive discount schemes that they often offer. Purchasing drugs at the right price is particularly important in relation to reimbursement and profit margins, as discussed later. Most wholesalers will deliver, if not daily, then several times a week and so it should not be necessary to keep huge stocks of drugs sitting on the dispensary shelves. Nevertheless, the average dispensary will still have stocks worth several thousands of pounds.

Labelling

The GMSC has issued the following advice to doctors concerning the labelling of containers for drugs. This advice also applies to drugs that are handed out from doctors' bags. The label should include the following:

- the name of the person to whom the medicinal product is to be administered
- the name, address and telephone number of the supplying doctor (or pharmacist)
- the date the medicines are dispensed
- the words 'keep out of reach of children', or words of similar meaning.

Unless drugs are supplied in original containers, they should be supplied in childproof containers unless the patient specifically requests otherwise. There are a number of commercial firms who will supply pre-printed labels for use by dispensing doctors so that the dispensary computer or labelling machine needs only to print on the details relevant to that particular preparation.

Reimbursement

This critically important aspect of dispensing is covered in Paragraphs 44.1– 44.5 of the Statement of Fees and Allowances (Red Book). Payments are made to doctors for the supply of drugs and appliances where they have been supplied and personally administered by prescribing or dispensing doctors to any patient in accordance with arrangements made under the relevant section of the NHS Acts, and to dispensing doctors where drugs or appliances have been supplied to patients on their dispensing lists or to temporary residents. Paragraph 44.2 spells out how the payments are made up.

44.2 Payments for drugs and appliances (other than for oxygen and oxygen therapy equipment – see Paragraph 44.3) shall be as follows:

i the basic price. This is the price as defined in Part II Clauses 8 and 11 of the Drug Tariff
less (except where the practitioner has been exempted under Paragraphs 44.7 or 44.8) a discount calculated in accordance with Paragraph 44/Schedule 1

ii an on-cost allowance of 10.55% of the basic price before deduction of any discount under Paragraph 44/Schedule 1

iii a container allowance of 3.8p per prescription

iv a dispensing fee as shown in Paragraph 44/Schedule 2

v an allowance in respect of VAT calculated in accordance with Paragraph 44.4

vi exceptional expenses as provided for in Part II Clause 12 of the Drug Tariff.

The total amount arrived at for the cost of each prescribed item is then subject to a discount that is periodically reviewed by the Department of Health and recognizes the fact that dispensing doctors are normally able to buy their supplies at less than the advertised price. This mechanism ensures that doctors are reimbursed only for what they have actually spent and do not gain unfair financial advantage from the 'pool system' of calculating and remunerating doctors' expenses.

In the case of doctors working in very remote areas and small practices, or where the number of patients on the dispensing list is very small, it may not be possible to obtain any discount on the advertised price. Indeed, they may have to pay more than the normal basic price. Special arrangements exist, described in Paragraph 44.8 of the SFA for reimbursement in these circumstances.

It is vitally important in a dispensing practice that every doctor always writes a prescription for any item supplied to a patient, in order that the practice can be reimbursed. In the case of non-dispensing patients it is still important that personal administration prescriptions are written and collected each month so that they can be sent off to the PPA so that the FHSA can reimburse the practice accordingly. Not only do the prescriptions have to be collected together, but each item has to be annotated with the name of the drug manufacturer, the pack size from which it was dispensed and the number of tablets or volume of medicine that was actually dispensed. At the end of each month dispensing doctors receive a payment 'on account' calculated by reference to their dispensing costs in that month in previous years; when the total value of the prescriptions actually dispensed for that month is worked out, usually two months later, a balancing payment is made.

As the 'Red Book' points out in Paragraph 44.12, it is critically important, in order to ensure that the annual survey of practitioners' practice expenses carried out by the Inland Revenue is as accurate as possible, that doctors ensure that their actual expenditure on drugs and appliances, i.e. the amounts they pay their suppliers, is shown gross in their accounts and not netted out after taking into account reimbursement they have received.

The rate of discount that is applied to the basic price is subject to a sliding scale based on the total basic price of all prescriptions submitted by a doctor or practice in any given month. Similarly, the dispensing fees payable are on a sliding scale related to the actual number of prescriptions submitted for pricing, and range from 88.1p per prescription, decreasing as the number of prescriptions dispensed increases.

Ordering stock and stock control

Modern technology has made the ordering of drug supplies much easier. Most wholesalers now use bar codes or numerical identifiers for most products and orders can be quickly entered into a small computer terminal in the dispensary and then transmitted via a modem to the wholesaler's own computer. Dispensary staff should be trained to ensure that whenever they become aware of supplies of a particular product running low they should order a new supply. In busy dispensaries, where the rate of use of commonly prescribed items remains fairly consistent, it may be possible to arrange for 'standing order' deliveries to be made.

Product liability

The law relating to product liability is a confusing mixture of rules, and the extent of the implications for GPs is not always clear. The law affects all situations in which products are supplied to patients directly. The effect of the law is such that, if a person suffers damage as a result of a defective product, it is no longer necessary to prove negligence, but only that the product was defective and the damage was a result of the defect in that product. The liability will generally fall on the manufacturer or the importer of the finished product into the country. However, in order to give the claimant a clear route of action, liability will fall on any supplier who cannot identify someone further up the chain of supply. A doctor supplying medicines must ensure that the manufacturer or importer is identifiable, otherwise the doctor will be deemed to be the producer and liable for any damage resulting from the product. Following the above guidance issued by the GMSC should ensure that doctors will not fall foul of the product liability laws.

Accurate records, such as invoices and the source of supply of all medicines and drugs, should be retained for a period of eleven years.

The product liability legislation imposes certain obligations on dispensing doctors. In the case of products supplied in their original packs, the doctor needs to be able to demonstrate from his records the name and address of the supplier from whom he obtained the drugs that he has dispensed. In the case of products that are supplied in small quantities from larger containers, i.e. 'broken bulk' supplies, the dispensing doctor should keep records of the batch number, the date of supply, the supplier and the manufacturer. Once again, guidance on this complex subject is available from the GMSC.

Practice formulary

The other piece of documentation that dispensing practices would be well advised to have is a written practice formulary. This should ensure that the members of the practice prescribe from that formulary and that the dispenser knows which products to stock as a matter of course and which products are only ordered in on a special 'one-off' basis. It helps to avoid duplicating stock and to ensure that in each therapeutic group a reasonable choice of drugs is available.

Prescription fees

Dispensing doctors are responsible for collecting prescription fees from those patients who are eligible to pay them. This is a somewhat irksome task, as the doctor is acting as an unpaid tax collector. Patients who claim they are exempt from payment should be asked to endorse the back of the prescription form to that effect. It is not part of the doctor's responsibility to challenge their claimed exemption, but the doctor does have to account for the prescription fees he has collected. Most FHSAs now require doctors to submit a statement at the end of each month stating how much they have collected in prescription fees, and this is paid by the practice into its own account, with a corresponding amount being deducted from the reimbursement that the FHSA sends at the end of each month.

Dealing with unwanted and out-of-date medicines

Many patients will return their unwanted medicines to the doctor's dispensary for safe disposal. In addition, the dispensary staff may, from time to time, find that some stocks have run out of date and have to be disposed of. Careful monitoring by the dispensary staff should minimize this and in many instances drugs nearing the end of their shelf life can be returned to the wholesaler or manufacturer and reimbursements made. Most FHSAs have in place a system for the collection and safe disposal of unwanted drugs and dispensing doctors should familiarize themselves with these arrangements.

Patient information cards and enquiries

As the source of supply of drugs and medicines to patients, dispensing doctors and their staff will inevitably have to answer the questions asked by patients about the medicines they are going to take. This requires familiarity with the appearance of the drugs, being able to give advice about when to take them and a knowledge of their interactions with other drugs and over-the-counter remedies. Dispensing doctors will be responsible for supplying drug information cards and for ensuring patients understand any special warnings in relation to a particular product.

Benefits of dispensing

There is no doubt that dispensing by doctors is a service highly valued by patients. It provides them with an immediate source of supply for their drugs 24 hours a day, seven days a week. It is also convenient for them, particularly in isolated rural areas. It enables the dispensing doctor to become familiar with the appearance of the drugs that he is asking his patients to take, and the actual process of dispensing and supplying medicines is an added interest to the practice of medicine. Whilst the service is there primarily for the benefit of patients, it does also provide a useful source of income to doctors in country practices, many of whom have smaller than average lists and high overheads. The income from dispensing helps them to maintain an overall income level comparable with that of their urban colleagues, and goes some way to compensate them for the loss of earning opportunities available to doctors in more urban areas.

14   The electronic *British National Formulary*

Anne B Prasad

This chapter deals with the development of the *BNF* as an electronic drug information data base and the significance of this to the broader field of decision support. Mention will also be made of some of the additional features that could spring from this, and of the future potential of electronic libraries.

The *BNF* has a pivotal role in general practice prescribing and it is now some years ago since we recognized that it could act as an authoritative electronic drug information source, able not only to cover details of products on the UK market, but also to provide critical insight into their respective merits. The ideal decision-support system would link this drug information with other practical aspects of prescribing, including patient records, local prescribing policies and budget control.

During the years leading up to the electronic development, the presentation of the *BNF* data was rationalized into as appropriate an order as possible for the rigorous requirements of computers. At the same time, however, a decision was taken that the *BNF* should appear on screen in its familiar pocket-book format. The editorial message should not be distorted to suit the requirements of the software.

It has taken a long time to achieve the breadth of coverage of the data contained in the *BNF* and the aim was to take it in its entirety to the electronic screen. It was considered that the users of electronic systems would appreciate seeing on screen the version with which they had long grown familiar. This account of the electronic *BNF* therefore starts with a brief step into the past of the paper version and a brief account of its evolution to the dominant role which it occupies in UK drug information today.

History of the *BNF*

The *BNF* has its roots in the health insurance formularies of the 1930s. Following the outbreak of the Second World War these were united into a *National War Formulary* which provided formulas incorporating substitutes for scarce imported ingredients. Although this was only fifty years ago, few of these ingredients remain in the *BNF* of today.

The first *BNF* proper was produced in 1949 following the inception of the National Health Service. Coverage in this early *BNF* was highly selective and by the time the last of these had been produced, covering the period 1976–8, a need had been detected for a more comprehensive formulary incorporating a much wider range of preparations and providing informed advice on their relative merits. A new style of *BNF* was therefore designed to respond to these needs. Whereas the old *BNF* had been selective and revised once every two to three years only, this new *BNF* would be comprehensive, with a new edition every six months.

Box 14.1: Aims of the *BNF*

- effective, safe, and economical drug utilization
- education.

The first of these new *BNFs* was published in 1981. The *BNF* of today aims to be an up-to-date pocket book for rapid reference by practising doctors and pharmacists, and to encourage safe, rational and cost-effective prescribing. It is also widely used by nurses and other health care professionals and is an educational tool for medical and pharmacy students. Dentists receive a special *Dental Practitioners' Formulary* bound with the *BNF*, which is revised every two years and which includes advice for the specialized requirements of dentists. Recently a pilot version of a *Nurse Prescribers' Formulary* has been produced; designed to be bound into the main *BNF*, it contains advice for the new generation of nurse prescribers.

Authority of the *BNF*

The *BNF* is published jointly by the British Medical Association and the Royal Pharmaceutical Society. One of its most important features is that it is an independent publication, published by and for the professions. It is produced under the authority of a Joint Formulary Committee that comprises representatives from the two professions and from key sections of the Department of Health. The Chairman of the Joint Formulary Committee is appointed by the two professions.

While the information in the drug monographs reflects the data sheets (and hence the product licences), the notes in the different sections of the *BNF* are based on the advice of practising expert clinicians. As well as expert advisers for each section, the *BNF* also has expert advisers in paediatrics and in geriatrics.

Box 14.2: Sources of *BNF* data

- expert advisers
- government and WHO publications
- data sheets
- journals and text books
- professional and legal guidelines.

In addition, the notes in the *BNF* are subject to continuous internal review against the published literature. Input from many other sources, such as the Joint Committee on Vaccination and Immunization, is also incorporated into the *BNF*. As part of the overall review process, a copy of each edition is sent to all companies whose products are included in the *BNF*.

Information in the *BNF* takes account of:

- standard nomenclature
- legal and professional requirements
- the requirements of the licensing authority
- clinical practice.

Thus, the *BNF* integrates legal and clinical requirements. Integration of these different requirements entails pro-active editing and the continuous advice of experts from many fields.

The scope of the *BNF*

The *BNF* includes advice on:

- dosage, cautions, contra-indications, side-effects, interactions, hepatic and renal impairment, pregnancy and breast-feeding.

In addition, clinical guidelines cover areas such as:

- controlled drugs, children, the elderly, terminal care, management of poisoning.

Above all, clinical advice is available for most common medical conditions, supplemented by consensus views in key areas such as:

- hypertension, asthma, antipsychotic therapy, prophylaxis of endocarditis, pulmonary tuberculosis, prophylaxis and treatment of malaria, family planning, vaccination.

Finally, authoritative guidance is provided in areas of special concern or controversy such as:

- anaphylaxis, benzodiazepine withdrawal, appetite control, hormone replacement therapy, oral rehydration, topical corticosteroids.

The aim of an electronic version of the *BNF* would be to make all this information available at the press of a button.

Why go electronic?

Many medical editors have recognized the advantages of presenting their books and journals in an electronic format. No matter how wise the advice or how attractively presented the arguments in the paper version, all is to no avail if today's health care workers are obliged by pressure of time to resort to the electronic screen as a major source of guidance. Moreover, it was clear that an electronic version of the *BNF* would not only complement the paper version, but would also be able to provide additional features outside the remit of its pocket-book format.

The phase I development of the electronic *BNF*

The development of the electronic *BNF* is being undertaken in two phases:

- phase I (which has now been completed)
- phase II (which is now underway and is due for completion in early 1996).

Phase I of the development of the electronic *BNF* has provided the following:

- an in-house data base in a simple format which can be managed and updated by the editorial staff (from which the paper version can be typeset and printed)

- an electronic version suitable for sale on disk or CD-ROM as a stand-alone system (the software displaying on screen the same layout as the book)

- a simple data base version suitable for developers to integrate into their own practice software systems.

The procedure for the phase I development

Quartet Software Ltd, a company that includes a desktop publishing expert and two general practitioners with decision support expertise, was employed to design the software. These skills responded to our two main requirements. It was essential to remember that, at the same time as an electronic version was produced, the paper version was still needed. An excellent rapport was established with Quartet that was to stand firm throughout the demanding times to follow.

The intricacies of the task soon became apparent. The first hurdle was to strip the existing typesetting file of its electronic codes to meet the more rigorous logic required for the purposes of a fully-fledged data base. Many of the typesetting commands would need to be replaced: italics, bolds, capitals and word breaks would need to be rechecked and even paragraph breaks might sometimes go missing. Checking procedures were established to identify and correct these.

One constraint was that the classification could not be amended into what might appear to be a more logical order. Too many sources, including the PPA, the Read codes, and a host of hospital and general practice formularies, relied on it. Moreover, under no circumstances could the demands of the software be allowed to intrude upon the readability of the book. The aim throughout was that the electronic *BNF* should incorporate all the advantages of the existing pocket book version and go a step further. Happily, it was no problem to elicit an underlying logical scaffolding that could be used to support the data on the computer.

Early work on the database

The months passed and many problems were resolved. In particular, the seemingly innumerable variations in the style were reviewed. Gradually, logical sets emerged and the new database was able to assert its authority over the unruly data. Finally, the database reflecting *BNF* No. 26 was delivered, the small tape seeming a modest exterior for the impact it would have on the production procedures. New safety systems were in place, as was a special audit trail.

Attempts had been made to anticipate and cover all eventualities, but still the new database could not be tested immediately because, by now, the production of the next *BNF*, using standard typesetting methods, was well advanced. At last, in March 1994, the *BNF*'s electronic days began, when the database was updated to reflect the newly published *BNF* No. 27.

It is a big job to move over quarter of a million words from a typographical file to a database. Security was the key issue and involved countless hours of proofreading. Above all else, it was vital to ensure that during the transfer nothing had been lost or jumbled. During the conversion, two full parallel proofreadings were carried out between *BNF* No. 26 and *BNF* No. 27, and a further two were required between *BNF* No. 27 and *BNF* No. 28.

Eventually, much as a room that has been pulled apart for redecoration is finally restored to order again, so did the familiar *BNF* re-emerge. *BNF* No. 28 was the first edition to be published entirely from the new database intact, checked and validated.

Advantages of the electronic *BNF*

Undoubtedly from the point of view of its production, the chief advantage of the electronic *BNF* is that additions can be made at a much later stage than was possible previously. Another advantage is that the presentation can be adjusted more easily. No matter how valuable, however, these advantages would not in themselves have justified the creation of a database. By far the most important advantage of the electronic *BNF* will be improved accessibility for the user.

The phase I product

On screen the electronic *BNF* looks similar to the pocket book version. The user can view the columns on the computer screen and browse through the data using search commands available through a program that allows the text to be viewed in 'column image' form. While the visual image will be similar to the book form, the search facility will enable the user to extract information more rapidly than from the paper version. There is an index, but many people may prefer to access the data through the contents list, jumping into chapters, sections, drug monographs and preparations at will. An important feature is that it is possible to jump to the section on interactions. It is in colour and hazardous interactions are preceded by red flags, while the less hazardous interactions are preceded by yellow flags.

The Phase I version of the electronic *BNF* should already be a valuable support for the prescriber. Much more is planned, however, and phase II, now underway, involves detailed structuring of the information to allow the database to operate as part of an intelligent decision-support and prescribing tool.

Phase II development of the electronic *BNF*

The phase II electronic *BNF* will provide links to patient records so that system developers can integrate the resulting knowledge system into their own practice software. The data will continue to appear on the screen in the *BNF* column format, but the text will be embedded with many electronic codes so that suppliers can use it to respond intelligently to details in a patient's records. In order that the natural language of the book can still be used, a set of standard *BNF* terms has been developed to identify the natural language knowledge entities in the *BNF*. It is hoped that mapping these standard *BNF* terms to the equivalent Read codes will provide the *BNF* with an intelligent link to patient records. The advice will still be in column format, but it will be an intelligent and responsive column with the relevant section highlighted. It is hoped that enabling the prescriber to view the specific warning in the context of the more general warnings will provide an intuitive sense of the overall profile of side-effects.

The set of standard *BNF* terms that will link to natural language knowledge entities in the *BNF* for use within decision-support systems can be viewed as an intricate extension of the existing *BNF* classification system and will unify the existing classification with the back-of-the-book index terms. The *BNF* classification system is already used widely throughout the country free of copyright, and we intend to make our extended classification system available similarly. The data and format will, however, remain copyright.

Applications of the phase II electronic *BNF*

The major application of the phase II electronic *BNF* is as a tool for prescribing support. It is also hoped that it may be appropriate for use as a key knowledge base for the broader field of extended decision support. Security is seen as a major issue and even in the early stages it is planned to introduce security checks to support the prescriber. Similar in-built security checks are planned to support dispensing. There is no doubt that in-built safety features are essential. Such safety checks need not impose themselves upon the prescriber. In order to prevent them from being too intrusive there are plans to permit the *BNF* database to be used for various research projects whose aim will be to obtain feedback on exactly what level of drug knowledge support is needed for prescribers.

Another application of the phase II version of the electronic *BNF* is to incorporate it within an electronic 'bookshelf' providing a range of electronic books. Soon the prescriber should be able to move swiftly from clinical textbook to drug bulletin to pocket book. An electronically-stored range of reference books, linked by a common electronic index for access from different points of view and at different levels of complexity, is at last a feasible electronic tool. It is envisaged that the *BNF* will be able to carry its pocket-book role into such a library. The electronic *BNF* may also soon act as a host to the papers and documents that are reflected in its guidelines. It would be reassuring to have background sources to check when dealing with important issues affecting overall prescribing policy.

Cost is an important issue in prescribing and bar charts can be a great help. Space has been at too much of a premium to permit inclusion of bar charts in the pocket book version, but there will be no problem in the database. Algorithms would even permit the creation of customized bar charts. These bar charts could be printed out for study or discussion.

Another application of the phase II electronic *BNF* should be to provide simple links for general practice formularies. Rather than create a formulary only to discover with a subsequent edition of the *BNF* that it is out of date, it would be simpler to create a customized formulary with links to the electronic *BNF*. Thus, the *BNF* hopes to provide support for general practice and other formularies.

Much of the *BNF* amounts to a distillation or interpretation of the data sheets. There is a need for a rapid link into the data sheets so that, when taking difficult decisions, prescribers may have the confidence of having checked more than one source. To this end the *BNF* standard terms could be a practical link, which need not obviate links with other systems (such as the Medicine Control Agency's ADROIT system).

The *BNF* already reflects many authoritative consensus guidelines and has now started to carry the views of expert groups in difficult or controversial areas (such as high-dose antipsychotic therapy). There is no reason why the electronic version should not provide further details of such groups (such as addresses of counselling centres).

Soon, medicines will be supplied with patient information leaflets. It is not a function of the *BNF* to generate these. However, as patients develop more insight into medical care they may require additional documents explaining a condition in the context of its overall management. The electronic *BNF* could host such documents which could be printed out in the surgery.

Conclusion

The electronic *BNF* will be able to act as a knowledge base for prescribing and decision support. It is hoped that the future will see the evolution of many companion electronic books which will gradually link into a library to provide the full range of decision support for the prescriber. Other applications of the electronic *BNF* will be its ability to host useful supplementary documents and to provide support for the development of local formularies.

15 Drug trials in general practice

Michael Drury

Introduction

General practitioners are frequently invited to participate in the trial of a drug, involving their own patients. Apart from the ethical issues, there are concerns surrounding such trials that merit consideration. They are often complex and always time-consuming, and, given that few doctors are now looking for more work, serious questions need to be asked about their scientific value, the purpose behind some requests to participate, and the desirability of doctors, already hard-pushed, spending time and resources upon such activities. Furthermore, if good medical practice is to be based on the results of such studies, can they be carried out to a sufficiently high, scientific standard in the context of a busy service practice?

Why carry out trials in general practice?

Patients who are in hospital are in much more controlled situations. Their drugs are issued regularly and in reliable quantities, baseline measurements of weight, pulse and blood pressure are routinely recorded and measurements of heart, lung, liver and kidney function can be obtained with ease. Diet and exercise can be carefully controlled so that variations can be limited and the situation is such that one may readily believe one is comparing like with like. These considerations may suggest that this is a better area for drug trials than the community. Outside hospital, people are much more autonomous and exposed to an unpredictable set of influences. They may attend when they are supposed to or they may not; they may take their drugs as directed or as they find convenient; and arranging sophisticated investigation is much more difficult.

A part of the reason for carrying out drug trials in the community is just this variability. Even though trials are often more difficult to do in this situation, it is important to understand how a patient and his drugs will interact in the real world; when they are eating or refraining from food, when they exercise and when they rest, and when they may be suffering from fatigue, colds, and all the other influences and pressures of daily living. Without this, a true picture of the risk/benefit of the drug may never be built up.

Whilst this is a very important reason for needing to carry out community trials, there are also other reasons. Some diseases are confined to, or mainly to be found in, patients who are ambulant and living in their own homes. This may include those attending out-patient departments, but there are diseases and problems that are rarely seen there. These are not only minor conditions such as the common cold, allergies, gastroenteritis or anxiety states, but also many major problems such as asthma, arthritis, depression and high blood pressure. Some drugs are given for long periods, such as oral contraceptives or drugs for chronic disease; and large numbers of patients may need to be observed for long periods to determine the efficacy or safety of the preparation – something that is best done in general practice.

There is one other factor, which arises from the structure of primary care in the UK. Because patients will, by and large, receive all their care from a single source and cannot 'shop around' for care, as they can in many other countries, it is possible to keep a much tighter record of all the events occurring to a patient whilst they are enrolled in a trial – with obvious benefit to the study. Indeed, the ability to carry out high-quality clinical trials is one reason for the strength of the pharmaceutical industry in the UK. On balance, there are strong reasons for as many GPs as possible to be involved in such trials.

It is worth pointing out some other benefits that patients and practices obtain from participating in trials. Patients who are recruited will often get a much more thorough examination and investigation than they otherwise would have done. Doctors may well find that at the end they know more about the patient and especially the disease than they previously did, so that other patients may benefit. Finally, doctors are reminded of the scientific method and may find their interest in research stimulated by this exercise.

There are, however, some quite formidable problems on the opposite side. The relationship between a patient and the doctor is often very personal and intense in general practice. This makes persuading patients much easier to accomplish but may leave the doctors with a sense of unease about their role as a persuader. When this means, as it almost always does, more time-consuming consultations involving travel, time off work, demands on other people and certain anxiety, the unease may be greater. The relative prevalence of the disease under study is another major problem. In most cases there will be only a few sufferers within an individual practice, say five to 20. Indeed, if there were more, the logistics of doing a study without disturbing and causing disadvantage to the care of other patients, would become too difficult. The fact that a study has to be carried out in a number of centres increases the problems of communication, co-ordination and audit. This can severely test the quality and reliability of the study and deserves special attention.

Phases of investigation of a new drug

The phases of investigation that a new drug has to pass through before it is licensed for routine prescription are complex. For every drug that emerges for clinical trial more than 20 compounds will have started but fallen by the way. Most of these will have undergone testing in animal models to determine such things as effect, dose and toxicity before the first phase of testing in a limited number of human volunteers takes place. Once this stage has generated enough data, patients will be needed in order to determine the effect of the drug upon the disease process under investigation. This stage, phase II, involves very limited numbers of patients in very rigorously-controlled and observed situations, and hence almost always hospital in-patients. General practice is never involved in studies at this level. In phase III studies, however, where several hundred or several thousand patients are required to obtain evidence of efficacy and safety, general practitioners are becoming more frequently involved.

All these studies take place before the drug can be licensed and marketed, and their aim is to produce data for consideration by the Medicines Control Agency or, in the USA, the Food and Drug Administration, whose task is to approve for licensing. Once this is achieved, phase IV studies may be required and these are predominantly carried out in general practice. They may look into matters such as different dosage schedules, new indications for

---

Box 15.1: Clinical developments of new drugs

Phase I   Clinical pharmacology in normal volunteers generating pharmacokinetic, metabolic and pharmacodynamic data

Phase II   Clinical investigation to confirm kinetics and dynamics in patients

Phase III   Formal therapeutic trials to establish efficacy and determine safety

Phase IV   Further formal trials, including comparative studies and PMS

an already licensed preparation or new formulations of the drug. They must be differentiated from post-marketing surveillance (PMS) which is usually concerned with the identification of adverse events occurring during the uncontrolled administration of the drug to thousands of patients.

What is a clinical trial?

Such trials have been around since biblical times, but the randomized controlled trial described and launched by Cochrane after the Second World War has now become the 'gold standard' for clinical trials. Before the advent of this technique, treatment groups were compared to historical controls or simultaneous controls, but observers found it difficult or impossible to distinguish change due to treatment from variations due to selection of patients. With careful design it is now possible, by random allocation of patients, to produce results that will stand up to statistical analysis.

Essential though random allocation to control and study groups is, there are other well-defined steps in protocol design that every doctor involved in trial work needs to understand. It is important that the clinician should be able to distinguish between good and bad studies: not only is it unethical to involve patients in a study that is incapable of producing a reliable answer, but whoever is paying for treatment – in the UK the NHS – may decline to support treatment that has not been shown to help more than harm or to be cost effective.

These steps in protocol design are set out below in the way they will appear in a well-designed protocol.

The question to be answered

Every trial should seek the answer to a question that is as simple as possible and is important. It should be capable of providing an answer that will stand up to analysis and will provide the patient with confidence that the treatment has a chance of success.

The patients to be studied

There should be an exact description of all the patients recruited to the study. This should include all the reasons for exclusion and the study result should detail the reasons for exclusions of each patient so that the reader can determine those to whom the conclusions did not apply.

The study design

The most common and simple design is a comparison of treatment with the study drug in a random group of patients with treatment of another random group given the current 'best buy' drug. A placebo may also be required in order to test 'no treatment' against any treatment if spontaneous recovery or change is to be assessed, but it would be unethical to use one where some treatment of proven value already exists. Sometimes more than one treatment, such as different doses of the same drug, can be tested within large groups, and sometimes cross-over studies can produce valuable data whilst keeping the number of patients relatively small. Unless there are clear reasons for doing otherwise, it is a *sine qua non* that all patients entered in a study should be included in the analysis. Some patients will probably be withdrawn during the course of the study, but they have to be included in the analysis otherwise serious skewing of the results may occur.

How long is the study to continue?

The length of a study is determined by the number of completed patients required to answer the question. It would be unethical to recruit more patients to a study than are required to give the answer, and this would certainly lead to questions being asked about whether there was an element of concealed marketing in the design. It is also important that a study which aims to affect the course of chronic disease but not to affect the cure should make clear what is to happen to patients who are on the study drug at the end of the trial. A patient who is benefitting from a study drug may reasonably be expected to have continuing access to the drug.

'Blinding' of patient and investigators

Double blinding has become a standard requirement of most controlled trials. It is usually obtained by having the study drug, the comparator drug and any dummy capsules required formulated identically. In order to get complete 'blinding', the random allocation, the patient, the doctor, the interpreter of investigations, the patients who are withdrawn and the statistician have all to be 'blinded'. If the chain is broken at any point, the patient concerned has to be withdrawn. A system for breaking the 'blinding' code has to be installed, since physicians treating the patient for co-existing disease will need to know what drugs are being administered.

Ethical considerations

Every trial on an NHS patient or involving NHS premises, staff or equipment requires ethical approval by a Local Research Ethics Committee (LREC). These have been set up in each health district in England and Wales and by health boards in Scotland. Their constitution has been established by the Department of Health, with eight to 12 members, of whom either the chairman or the vice-chairman should be a lay person. The other members will be drawn from hospital medical staff, nursing staff, general practitioners and two or more lay persons. Individuals do not represent specific group interests but are appointed as individuals 'of sound judgement'. Ethical approval is not a legal requirement but no NHS body will allow research to take place without it. Similarly, funding, publication and so on will usually require that the study has had ethical approval.

Factors that an ethics committee will consider include:

- objectives of the study and practical benefits envisaged

- study design

- nature of subjects involved, including controls and whether expenses are to be paid

- resource consequences for the NHS

- adequacy of researchers' resources

- things to be done to subjects and controls

- risks

- informed consent

- payment to researchers

- indemnity of subjects for injury

- quality assurance and publication.

This is not a comprehensive list but it reveals the main matters that will be considered. Often modifications will be sought and there may be at least two scrutinies of some protocols.

There is a particular problem associated with studies in general practice. Because of the nature of the study, these nearly always involve a number of practices, sometimes a hundred or more, spread over a wide geographical area and consequently falling under a number of ethics committees. Whilst it would be possible to obtain ethical approval from all the committees the difficulties in a large national study are very great. Apart from the cost of submitting nearly 2000 copies of the protocol, some committees require investigators to attend whilst others do not. Clearly the scientific detail of a study has to be identical wherever the study is done if data are to be capable of aggregation, but if different alterations are required by different committees, this can be destroyed. This problem is currently under consideration and it looks as if there will be a system by which the science is reviewed by a single 'expert' committee, leaving local committees with the responsibility of ensuring that there are no unconsidered local issues.

Taking part in a clinical trial

Before agreeing to take part in a clinical trial you should understand that this is not to be undertaken lightly. It requires a high degree of commitment from you, the patients and others, such as practice nurses or partners, who may be involved. Protocols need to be followed meticulously and nothing that should be done can be missed out. The integrity of the trial depends upon the reliability of all the data used. Estimating, guessing or making up data after the event is a serious breach of trust, indeed so serious that several doctors have now been found guilty of serious professional misconduct for doing this and removed from the Medical Register for falsification of data. It is important when investigations, such as renal function tests, are part of the study, that not only are the results accurately entered on to forms but that the source documents are retained for checking. It is thus important to be quite realistic about the time involved and to be certain that you, and other members of the practice who may be involved, can do so without difficulty.

The second requirement is to be certain you actually want to take part. It is important to feel that you and patients will benefit and that you will find it stimulating. There needs to be at least an intellectual reward for taking part. With most studies payment for general practitioners is, reasonably, properly costed, but a trial should not be seen as a way of making money. It is a way of making a contribution to the basis of good-quality patient care and this must be its own reward. Payment, when made, is based on an estimate of the cost to the practitioner of doing work above and beyond the care of the patient, and is therefore quite separate from NHS earnings. Payment is not an essential ingredient and many important national studies, such as the oral contraceptive study of the Royal College of General Practitioners, ran for many years without any payment at all. In such studies it is sufficient for doctors to believe it is an important study designed to answer questions relevant to patient care.

The third requirement is to estimate reliably the number of patients you can bring to the study from your practice. It is a well known 'law' of research that as soon as you begin to study a condition it disappears. You may feel, for instance, that you have many patients under your care with, say, multiple sclerosis and estimate that you can bring ten people into the study. By the time you have worked through them, discarding those who meet the exclusion criteria and those who do not want to be involved, you may be left with a very small fraction of the number you began with. Generally speaking, you would be wise to halve the number you estimate and consider yourself fortunate if you do not have to halve it again.

Remember also that the study has usually been designed by someone else. It is someone else's baby and, whilst they may be wildly enthusiastic about their offspring, to you it will seem just another baby; maintaining your enthusiasm throughout is difficult but necessary. It is very important to take part in any meetings, particularly pre-trial briefings that take place. If you do not understand the study well at the beginning, muddle will ensue; and if practice nurses are to participate they should be full members and attend all meetings too. The trial co-ordinator will help by keeping participants aware of the state of play. In the same way, it is very important that someone within the practice keeps all those who are involved well informed and maintains the drive to complete the study speedily and accurately.

Post-marketing surveillance

Strictly speaking, PMS is not a clinical trial and most such studies do not require approval by an ethics committee. The objective of PMS is to contribute to the safety profile of a licensed drug by reporting all the adverse events occurring to a patient who has been prescribed the drug under surveillance in the normal way. In the better studies, patients are recruited from prescriptions that have been issued some time before: doctors are asked to identify all adverse happenings in the months after first prescription. This avoids the possibility of bias at the time of recruitment. The Drug

Surveillance Unit at Southampton has an enviable track record for such studies; it depends heavily upon a high response from doctors who have prescribed. In the author's view, participation in such studies, or notification *via* the Yellow Card system, is not an option for doctors to take or leave, but part of one's professional responsibility.

Questions to be answered before taking part in a clinical trial

- Has the practice the time, space and resources to take part?
- Have we the motivation to take part? Shall we enjoy it?
- Can we recruit the subjects?
- Is the study important and are the aims well set out?
- Is the protocol clear and precise?
- Has ethical approval been obtained?
- Are the financial arrangements agreed?

Further reading

Drury M. (1993) Clinical trials of drugs in general practice. *Prescribers' Journal,* **33:** 8–15.
Inman W H W (ed). (1986) *Monitoring for Drug Safety* (2nd edn). MTP Press Ltd, Lancaster.
Symposium (1991): Drug development and clinical trials. *Prescribers' Journal,* **31:** 219–57.

16 Community pharmacists

Ravi S Gidar

The world is changing for community pharmacists. Their university degree course, which is soon to be lengthened from three years to four, is nowadays followed by a year of pre-registration training under an approved trainer, and registration is granted only after an examination set by the Royal Pharmaceutical Society of Great Britain. When they enter community practice they increasingly undertake continuing education. Current topics in workshops include: GP formulary development, child health, incontinence, transfer of care, home visits and repeat prescribing. It is likely that continuing education will become mandatory in the future. They want to have a new kind of professional life that will recognize the extent and nature of their training commitment.

Dispensing prescribed medicines and advising on their safe use remains the community pharmacist's main role, but the process of dispensing has become more complex: it involves checking the dosage, and the possibility of interactions with other drugs being taken, or with alcohol, and, increasingly, entering new information on to a computerized patient medication record. Drugs must have suitable cautionary labelling, and advice on how to take or use the medication must be given to the patient or the patient's representative.

Other services that may be provided include:

- a domiciliary oxygen service
- a display of health education literature
- advice to residential and nursing homes
- out-of-hours service
- a needle exchange system
- home visits
- health promotion, e.g. smoking cessation
- screening tests, e.g. blood pressure recording.

Community pharmacists see their future in terms of involvement in patient care, coupled with a high level of service. They are likely to work within or adjacent to GPs' surgeries, or to be sited within large stores or supermarkets.

Along with the drive to enlarge the role of pharmaceutical care, there is a desire to become more involved with primary health care teams – not only the doctors, but also the nurses, physiotherapists, dieticians and other members of the team. This is happening at a time when many practices are trying to improve their prescribing and looking for ways of constraining its costs safely. Community pharmacists can provide a resource for helping them to achieve these goals, and this was one of the recommendations of the Joint Working Party on the Future for Community Pharmacy in 1992.

A few years ago, when the author worked in West Sussex, the FHSA was keen to encourage links between GPs and community pharmacists. When incentive schemes for GP prescribing were introduced, it made regular meetings at least once a quarter, between practices and community pharmacists, one of the criteria that would be taken into account.

Local pharmacists were invited to meetings to train them for this new venture, which was modelled on work being done in Holland. The first task was to establish their training needs. Most of them thought that they required better communication skills as well as some form of clinical training, and help was given by both FHSA pharmaceutical advisers and postgraduate tutors in pharmacy. PACT analysis was also an important part of the training.

When the pharmacists started making their visits to practices it was found that they became increasingly involved in prescribing issues. Among the areas in which they were able to help were:

- advice on generic availability – the GPs were often not aware of the new generic preparations coming on the market
- pack sizes, packaging and alternative formulations
- Over-the-counter products, especially those that were being deregulated from prescription-only status
- improving patient compliance
- providing feedback on patients' attitude
- using the Drug Tariff
- PACT analysis
- repeat prescribing, including the duration of prescriptions
- reviews of patients' medication
- co-ordinating changes
- the development of formularies.

The GPs reported that they found the meetings interesting and informative; the community pharmacists said they learned a great deal and valued the closer working relationships that developed – a great improvement on just contacting a GP about some error of dosage or quantity on a prescription. The GPs also said that the community pharmacists were particularly valuable when they wanted to construct their own formularies – they tended to understand local prescribing habits better than the FHSA advisers did.

One of the main outcomes observed was an increase in the number of patients referred by the pharmacist to the GP, and by the GP to the pharmacist. Greater awareness of each others' situation and roles thus seemed to promote more effective and efficient primary care, as well as leading to more rational and economical prescribing.

One interesting effect of the visits was that they increased communication between partners in the same practice. One practice had four partners who never held any formal clinical meetings and who seemed to be totally isolated from each other. The regular, informal discussions initiated by the pharmacist over coffee and lunch eventually led to them developing a common philosophy of consulting style and drug usage, with the pharmacist regarded as part of the practice team.

This project was funded by the FHSA, and the community pharmacists were paid a nominal sum for their visits. The scheme was regarded as a great success, both in improving the care of patients and in containing prescribing costs. It certainly did a great deal to produce a closer relationship between the two professions. Community pharmacists welcome this new kind of role and the challenge it offers them – they hope that the NHS will see the value of funding it.

Further reading

Anon. (1986) A Report to the Nuffield Foundation. Pharmaceutical Journal, 236: 348–55.
Anon. (1992) Pharmaceutical care: the future for community pharmacy. Report of the Joint Working Party. Pharmaceutical Journal, 248: 541–4.
National Audit Office Report. (1992) Community pharmacists in England. HMSO, London.

17 Information pharmacists

Nicholas W Hough

Introduction

This chapter is entitled Information Pharmacists, but it is not just those with specialist skills in the NHS drug information (DI) service who fit this description. Pharmacists working in a variety of environments are increasingly becoming involved in providing information and advice about medicines and prescribing. There are new roles emerging for community pharmacists and most FHSAs employ pharmaceutical advisers whose responsibilities overlap with those of medical prescribing advisers.

In order to appreciate why pharmacists have found themselves so involved in information provision, it is necessary to consider the reasons why GPs require advice on medicines and prescribing. A basic understanding and some facts about the pharmaceutical 'market place' will highlight the importance of access to a variety of sources of drug information in today's NHS.

The role of pharmacists in providing information and advice about medicines and prescribing

The traditional role of the pharmacist has been the preparation and dispensing of medicines according to the prescriber's instructions, ensuring patient safety by acting as a safeguard against prescription errors, and advising patients on the correct use of their medicines. However, the training of pharmacists gives them the unique combination of a comprehensive knowledge and understanding of the actions and uses of drugs in relieving, curing or preventing illness, and also those aspects of pharmaceutical formulation that may affect a patient's response to drug treatment.

Specialization within the profession has occurred and 'drug information pharmacists' are employed by NHS drug information centres throughout the UK. Initiatives promoted by the Department of Health to monitor and manage prescribing in general practice have led to the appointment of FHSA pharmaceutical advisers. The traditional pharmacist mentioned earlier has also been encouraged to adopt a new role, relying less on the mechanical process of dispensing (which nowadays is increasingly a matter of re-packaging or re-labelling 'ready to use' products manufactured by the pharmaceutical industry) and more on the provision of professional advice to both prescribers and patients.

Community pharmacists

In many instances in the past, the main contact between community pharmacists and GPs has come from those occasions when there is a problem with a prescription. Although this is a very important process, it is not the most effective way to make use of their combined skills. Over the last three or four years, perhaps because of the introduction of the Indicative Prescribing Scheme (IPS), circumstances have begun to change. Opportunities have arisen for the two professions to work more closely alongside each other, (Chapter 16), and there is a greater need for sharing information about the use of medicines in the community. Improving Prescribing, the Department of Health's 1990 working paper that introduced the IPS, highlights several areas of common interest, including developing practice formularies and treatment protocols, encouraging generic prescribing, interpreting PACT data, and self audit of prescribing (see Box 17.1).

Whilst these are also the responsibility of FHSA prescribing advisers, community pharmacists are often better placed and more familiar with their local GPs' prescribing. Pharmacists have also regular personal contact with many of the patients from local practices. Consequently, they gain a good understanding of the health care needs of patients and a valuable insight into how well they manage their medicines.

The pharmacist is particularly well qualified to comment on the range of drugs being prescribed: for example the number of similar agents from within a single therapeutic category, and to suggest ways in which this can be simplified. Prescribers will then be able to choose from a narrower range of drugs with which they will become more familiar. Reassurance about the source and quality of generic products, and guidance about those drugs or formulations where it is necessary to prescribe a specified brand-name medicine, can also be given.

On their own initiative and through schemes organized by some FHSAs, a number of community pharmacists attend practice meetings to discuss prescribing issues. To support and encourage them in this role, the national Centre for Postgraduate Pharmacy Education (CPPE) produces a series of distance learning packs covering prescribing in each of the major therapeutic categories. All community pharmacies also receive the

Box 17.1: Areas of mutual interest to GPs and pharmacists in promoting rational prescribing

Development of formularies:

- selection of first choice drugs within each therapeutic category
- review and update procedures
- policy for including/excluding new drugs, and for prescribing new drugs before this decision has been made
- appropriate use of novel/expensive drug delivery systems.

Advice on generic prescribing:

- identifying appropriate generic 'switches'
- reassurance about the quality and appearance of generic medicines
- recommendations concerning 'brandname'-only prescribing for specific products
- strategies to inform patients about prescribing generics.

Interpretation of PACT:

- identifying possible problem areas, e.g. unnecessarily wide range of drugs prescribed
- identifying suitable drugs for the formulary
- monitoring adherence to a formulary
- comparison with local averages to detect and explain variations or inconsistencies.

MeReC Bulletin, enabling them to be aware of information and advice that GPs receive.

Some (non-dispensing) fundholding practices have gone a stage further and employ a full-time or part-time pharmacist as a member of the practice team. Since fundholders need to stay within their prescribing budgets, this approach may be particularly useful because the pharmacist is well placed to identify wasteful prescribing. Patients also benefit because there is someone available to advise them about the correct use of medicines.

FHSA pharmaceutical advisers

The FHSA pharmaceutical adviser role developed in response to the Improving Prescribing initiative. The initial intention was that FHSAs should appoint full-time (or shared full-time) medical prescribing advisers, and it was expected that any pharmaceutical advice needed could be obtained from district pharmaceutical officers or local drug information centres.

However, it soon became apparent that there was a need for further assistance with the IPS. Partly, this was due to the fact that it required more than one person to manage prescribing issues from the FHSA perspective, but also because medical advisers took on new responsibilities arising from the revised GP contract that had recently been imposed.

The FHSA professional advisers 'team' comprising medical and pharmaceutical input is now fairly well established. The roles of the medical and pharmaceutical adviser are complementary, and there are significant advantages in bringing together their professional expertise at the FHSA level. For example, the pharmacist provides a source of immediate knowledge about the various pharmaceutical products on the market, and knows where to look for more detailed background information. The doctor, usually an ex-GP, has the first-hand experience of the factors that influence prescribing in primary care.

The pharmacists may be better qualified to interpret PACT data and to undertake formulary development, especially if they have had previous experience in hospital where formularies are almost universal. The doctors may be more able to contribute to the development of treatment protocols since these may encompass clinical considerations other than prescribing. There may also be occasions when it is less threatening for GPs to discuss their own prescribing with a pharmacist, rather than with an ex-colleague who has crossed the 'management line' and become an employee of the FHSA.

Drug information (DI) pharmacists

The NHS Drug Information (DI) Network has developed over a twenty year period since the first DI centres were established in the UK in the early 1970s. The network consists of unit (hospital), district and regionally based DI centres, staffed by pharmacists. Although recent NHS reforms have had some impact on their distribution and responsibilities, there are still around 200 centres throughout the UK. DI centres often have close links with their local FHSA prescribing advisers. In fact, many of today's pharmaceutical advisers have previously worked at one time or another in the DI network.

Pharmacists who have chosen a career in DI undertake extensive training which covers issues such as enquiry answering, sources of information, on-line literature searching, evaluation of clinical trials, and legal and ethical aspects of information services. Further details about the services that DI centres provide, and the function of the national DI network are discussed later in this chapter.

What sort of drug information do GPs need and why do they need it?

GPs need information and advice to guide them on appropriate drug selection (in terms of effectiveness and safety), to keep up to date with advances in drug therapy, and to enable them to make optimum use of NHS resources (see Box 17.2). The last is particularly important, because, as fundholders have begun to realise, a greater proportion of the NHS drugs bill is becoming subject to tighter budgetary control.

Prescribing costs do account for a significant identifiable proportion of NHS financial resources. It could be argued that the drugs bill should not be

---

Box 17.2: Reasons why GPs need access to independent sources of information and advice about medicines and prescribing

- In order to ensure that prescribing is rational, i.e. appropriate, safe, efficacious, and cost effective.

- Drug therapy can sometimes be complex and hazardous and there is a need to avoid and detect adverse effects and interactions.

- There is such a wide variety of products available and GPs can be familiar with only a relatively small proportion of them.

- To understand the place in therapy of new drugs, especially those with unfamiliar pharmacology or biotechnological products.

- The pressures of drug company promotion and the competition between manufacturers for prescribers' attention and loyalty.

- Prescribing by GPs is a common activity, the total costs of which account for a substantial proportion of NHS resources.

more singled out for particular attention than any other item of expenditure. Nevertheless, a constant 10% per year of NHS finance is accounted for by prescribing, amounting to more than £3 billion. Since about 80% of this is spent in primary care, GPs have responsibility for the manner in which considerable sums of money are used. Expressing it another way, the cost of the average GP's prescribing is equivalent to twice his or her annual salary.

GPs are faced with a wide range of patients, from those presenting with relatively simple medical conditions, to others with multiple or complex disease states. Prescribing for the latter can often be hazardous because of the increased potential for drug interactions and adverse effects. Accessible information and advice to avoid these complications or to identify them when they occur is obviously necessary.

The pace of change in medical practice, particularly where pharmaceuticals are concerned, can be rapid. Within a few years of qualifying, most GPs find that new treatments and pharmacological advances bear little resemblance to the content of their undergraduate training.

Pharmaceutical companies spend millions of pounds promoting their products, particularly new medicines. The reason for this is not hard to understand. For example, it is now estimated that the research and development costs involved in launching a new medicine are in excess of £100 million. With limited time available under patent protection for exclusive marketing rights, i.e. before generic alternatives erode profits, there is enormous pressure to exploit the potential market for new drugs fully.

As a result the companies need to win prescribers over to their new treatments, which in some instances offer only minor advantages over established drugs, or have not been adequately defined in terms of their appropriate place in therapy. Against a background of competing promotional claims it may be very difficult for GPs to make rational drug selections consistently. Drug company promotion tends to draw attention only to specific features or potential advantages of the products. There is a need for some form of overall independent assessment of the range of therapies available, and an indication of which are appropriate first choice drugs.

Despite the recently increased investment by the Department of Health in monitoring and controlling the NHS drugs bill, promotional expenditure by the pharmaceutical industry far exceeds the resources available to the NHS. Whilst there may be around 300 full-time equivalent FHSA prescribing advisers in post, the industry employs about 6000 medical representatives in the UK. It has been shown on a number of occasions that representatives are one of the main influences on prescribing. About £300–350 million is spent annually on promotional activities, or about £10 000 per GP. Clearly the industry wouldn't commit itself to such outlay if it were not producing some effect!

Thus, it is vitally important for GPs to have access to reliable information and advice to help them select the medicines that are best for their patients and also represent value for money for the NHS. This advice needs to be up to date, relevant, and independent of any vested interests.

What sources of information are available?

There is a variety of sources of information and advice about medicines and prescribing available to GPs apart from direct contact with the pharmaceutical profession. These include various reference sources and other publications provided by the Department of Health. Pharmacists with information skills and expertise in the evaluation of medical literature are involved in the production of some of these. The sources described here are those which are either non-promotional or non-commercial. Emphasis is placed on official, professional, or NHS publications, and drug information services; reference to the *British National Formulary* has been omitted because this is comprehensively covered in a separate chapter.

The *Drug and Therapeutics Bulletin* (*DTB*)

The *DTB* is published by the Consumers' Association, to which the Department of Health pays a bulk subscription on behalf of all doctors in England. It is very well established and started life over thirty years ago. For many years it was the only source of independent advice and information on medicines and prescribing available to GPs.

Recently it has undergone a change from a fortnightly four-page to a monthly eight-page format. It still covers a very broad subject range, much of which is relevant to general practice. Topics include new product reviews, updates on the treatment of specific conditions, and practical issues such as the use of formularies. Articles appearing in the *DTB* aim to present a consensus view, and the preparation of material includes a review process involving many specialists and GPs. The often forthright approach taken by the *DTB* means that it is highly respected by most doctors and pharmacists.

Prescribers' Journal (*PJ*)

PJ is an in-house publication from the Department of Health, which contains articles independently authored by experts in the relevant field. Its production is overseen by a committee of management, supported by an advisory panel of experts and clinical pharmacologists. It is published every two months, and like the *DTB* has been produced for over thirty years.

The content of the *PJ* is somewhat different to the *DTB* (and the *MeReC Bulletin*), in that subjects are usually dealt with in a slightly broader context, in which prescribing may be one of the most important elements. On occasions a whole 'symposium' issue is devoted to a particular concept or disease area, or a specific patient group. It also features articles about the safety profile of specific drugs or drug groups.

The *MeReC Bulletin* and related initiatives

The *MeReC Bulletin* is sent to all GPs in England and is published in a four-page format every month by the Medicines Resource Centre (MeReC), an initiative launched by the Department of Health in 1990. Similar centres have since been established in Scotland and Wales. MeReC's origins owe much to the NHS drug information network because the centre produces on a national scale what a number of DI centres have done locally for many years.

MeReC is staffed by pharmacists with DI experience, all of whom contribute to the preparation of published articles. All the material is produced in-house, but is subjected to review and comments from specialists in the relevant field, various medical and pharmaceutical advisers, and DI pharmacists. Although funded directly by the Department of Health, MeReC operates independently on a day-to-day basis, particularly with regard to the selection of topics and content of articles.

The range of subjects covered is similar to that of the *DTB*, including new product assessments, reviews of drugs within the same therapeutic category, and the treatment of common medical conditions. The main difference is that it is aimed solely at GPs, and the emphasis is on those therapeutic areas where most prescribing takes place. MeReC's aim is to provide clear advice on appropriate drug selection, whilst providing enough detail to explain the rationale behind its conclusions and recommendations.

Both the *MeReC Bulletin* and the *DTB* examine the validity of promotional claims, and attempt to counter any misplaced enthusiasm generated by the launch of new drugs, or new uses for existing products. Information is provided about how new treatments compare with established therapy, and whether benefits demonstrated in clinical trials are likely to be achieved in everyday clinical practice. When worthwhile developments are introduced, advice is provided on the kinds of patient who are most likely to benefit. This information is extremely important in view of the vigorous marketing that accompanies 'breakthrough' products, to ensure that new drugs are used appropriately, safely, and cost-effectively.

An important feature of MeReC is its working relationship with the national Medical Advisers' Support Centre (MASC) with which it is co-located in Liverpool. MASC provides FHSA prescribing advisers with education and training in therapeutics and management skills, and the content of their programme is usually closely linked with that of MeReC bulletins. As a result, professional advisers are more effectively able to discuss prescribing issues with GPs during practice visits. MeReC also receives direct feedback from advisers on the needs of GPs for prescribing advice, and this helps in planning future publications. A series of MeReC Briefings is also produced for the advisers, which provides more detailed background information to facilitate their discussions with GPs. The Briefings are freely available to GPs and from time to time are distributed by some FHSAs.

A recent development has been the inclusion in the new PACT reports of a review of a therapeutic topic in the centre pages. This usually covers an area where it is felt that further information and advice will help to promote rational drug use. Many of the topics are planned to coincide with MeReC's publications, so that important prescribing messages are reinforced. The new PACT report also contains data pertaining to the recipient's own prescribing patterns in the area of interest. This should enable GPs to examine their use of drugs in the light of current recommendations of what represents best practice.

The NHS drug information network

DI services are not provided solely for the hospital sector. Because the service is usually located in a hospital, more of its work may be generated by hospital doctors than by GPs, but it is and has always been the case that NHS DI services are available to all prescribers. Some GPs may still not be familiar with what their local DI centre can do for them – probably because they do not have enough time to establish regular contact. They may remember the service only in some dire emergency.

The term '**drug information**' covers both enquiry answering and initiatives designed to influence prescribing pro-actively, for example by means of bulletins, face-to-face practice visits, or educational outreach. The former usually means dealing with specific prescribing problems related to individual patients, whilst the latter are intended to encourage rational and cost-effective drug use across a range of therapeutic areas.

All DI centres provide a comprehensive enquiry answering service on any aspect of drug therapy; these are summarized in Box 17.3. Each centre maintains or subscribes to a wide range of information sources, including journals and electronic databases. There are usually local arrangements to refer the more complex enquiries, or those that can be answered only by reference to less widely available resources, to the larger centres.

Box 17.3: Drug information centres are able to provide information and advice in relation to the following types of enquiry:

- indication and choice of therapy, and any contra-indications
- adverse effects
- drugs in pregnancy and lactation
- drug interactions
- administration and dosage
- availability, supply and costs of medicines
- pharmacology and therapeutics
- formulation
- identification, for example foreign medicines, loose tablets etc.

Sometimes an enquiry may require purely factual information; on other occasions, advice or a recommendation on the choice of therapy is needed. DI pharmacists are increasingly involved in the latter, basing their information on their own experience, knowledge of the medical literature, and liaison with experts in the relevant field.

One method of improving and publicising the DI service amongst GPs is by way of active dissemination of information. A number of regional and unit-based centres produce and distribute local newsletters and bulletins to keep prescribers up to date with advances in therapeutics, and to address local prescribing problems. The regional centre in the former Mersey RHA has been active in this way for some fifteen years or so. It was partly because of this that the Medicines Resource Centre (MeReC) was established in Liverpool.

The co-ordination and delivery of services through a national network has been one of DI's most successful achievements. This has prevented duplication of effort and fostered collaboration between the centres. One result has been the specialist information and advisory services that are provided from a number of the larger centres (see Box 17.4).

Box 17.4: Specialist information and advisory services

Specialist information on each of the following subjects is held by one or other of the regional DI centres

Drugs in breast milk	The respective specialist regional centres usually answer all types of
Drugs in pregnancy	enquiry related to their own subject of interest.
Drugs in dentistry	Most have access to specialist
Alternative medicine	textbooks and journals, and some also have in-house databases of
Drugs in renal failure	relevant literature.
Toxicology and poisoning	In some cases the centre may have access to expert practitioners in the
Drugs in liver failure	relevant field or to speciality departments within their own
Drugs in AIDS	hospital.

Out of the collaboration has come the 'new product assessment scheme'. Each of the contributing centres is allocated the task of evaluating a new product which is either just about to be marketed or still awaiting the granting of a product licence. A standardized format for the presentation and content of the assessments has been developed, and once complete they are circulated between the participating centres.

For new drugs that are similar to those already available such assessments highlight whether the new 'molecule' offers any potential benefits over existing drugs. In the case of more complex therapies or completely new chemical entities, particularly products resulting from biotechnological research, a more detailed evaluation is required. This will attempt to define a place in therapy and determine, from clinical studies undertaken with the drug, the patients who are most likely to benefit.

It is now becoming apparent that the NHS needs to anticipate those advances in therapy that are likely to have major financial or resource implications. The inclusion of disease incidence and prevalence data, and an estimate of the expected uptake of the treatment, are increasingly regarded as a vital features of these assessments. Advance 'intelligence' of therapeutic breakthroughs is increasingly becoming an important role for NHS DI services.

18   Pharmacoeconomics

Rhiannon T Edwards

Introduction

Drug costs account for about 10% of total NHS spending. In primary care, the drug bill accounts for about 50% of costs. The bill for primary care prescribing in the NHS has been rising steadily for some years, but recently the rate of rise has sometimes been as high as 14%, when general inflation is only around 3% (Figure 18.1). Is this rising drug bill of concern only to government and interested economists? Or is it, and what is more, should it be, the concern of GPs?

Doctors and economists: the need for a dialogue

There is a fundamental difference between the perspectives of clinicians and health economists: when faced with questions of what is good for society or

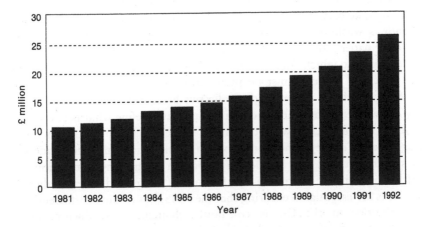

Figure 18.1 Total NHS spending on drugs 1981–92. (Source: *House of Commons Select Committee Enquiry into the NHS Drug Bill*, HMSO.)

good for a patient, doctors choose for their patient, as their training emphasizes, while to the economist, societal goals of efficiency and equity carry more weight.

The GP has a difficult dual role: on the one hand, he is the advocate of the individual patient, responding to the Hippocratic ethic that he must always do his best for that patient; on the other, he is also a guardian of the public purse, and acts in a gate-keeper role deciding which patients warrant spending more public money on. This gives doctors a role in rationing the use of NHS resources. Some doctors deny that they ever play such a role, but this is unrealistic: for instance, if faced with a waiting room full of patients, which doctor does not ration the amount of time he spends with each patient? (Resources refer to much more than just money – they include time and work also.) Given finite health care resources, if a doctor decides to use them to treat one patient, fewer are available to treat others (e.g. if you spend more time seeing one patient, you have less time to see everyone else). Health economists call this 'opportunity cost'.

The dilemma faced by doctors is illustrated in the BMA Handbook of Medical Ethics: 'As the resources within the NHS are limited, the doctor has a general duty to advise on their equitable allocation and efficient utilization. This duty is subordinate to his professional duty to the individual who seeks his professional advice'. So the BMA puts the needs of the individual patient ahead of the public good, and most doctors would agree with this – but there is clearly a tension between the two.

Some doctors regard it as totally unethical to consider costs in treating patients, but this does not stand up to much thought. If a doctor does not consider costs, he may be treating a patient inefficiently, and using resources inefficiently is wasteful: it cannot be ethical to waste scarce resources and deprive other patients of their value. This is not to suggest that efficiency is the highest endpoint to which doctors can aspire in their treatment – compassion for the individual patient must be prized also. The tensions between the needs of the individual patient and a collective body of patients are clear.

How can we begin to resolve these difficulties, and define what is effective and efficient treatment, i.e. what treatments work and what treatments are the best value for money? These will not be the only questions that decide a doctor's treatment, but they should play a part in the making of decisions.

Health economics and economic evaluations of drugs and other medical interventions are essential in ensuring that the NHS uses resources efficiently. General practice in the UK is constantly changing, and doctors are increasingly aware of the need to consider economic questions, and acknowledging a professional duty to ensure that clinical and rationing decisions remain in the hands of doctors, with the health economist in a supporting role. It is perhaps unreasonable to expect the individual doctor to make decisions about rationing, but it is reasonable that he should operate within the well publicized rationing guidelines that result from consultation between government, the profession and the public.

In the future, the development of training in health economics for medical students should be encouraged. Doctors and health economists must speak to one another, learning one another's jargon and hence beginning to see one another's viewpoint. This requires a compromise both for the doctors' Hippocratic ethic and the health economists' utilitarianism.

GPs, particularly those who are fundholders, are beginning to take a more societal view of the patient population for whose health they are responsible. Many are taking a growing interest in the economic evidence on the relative cost effectiveness of different drugs published in the pharmacoeconomic literature and wider clinical literature. Perhaps with a view to following Canada and Australia, which require economic evidence for the licensing of new pharmaceutical products, the UK pharmaceutical industry is being encouraged to provide not only evidence of the efficacy of their new products but also of their costeffectiveness. GPs, encouraged to draw up and adopt practice and district formularies, will need an understanding of the perspective, methods and jargon of economic evaluation to interpret the findings of published studies and to weigh up the economic arguments entering pharmaceutical advertising. It is hoped that this chapter can provide the reader with an insight into the perspective, terminology and methodology of health economics and can provide a first step towards such a common dialogue between doctors and economists.

Pharmacoeconomics and health economics

Pharmacoeconomics is the application of methods of economic evaluation, developed by health economists, to the appraisal of pharmaceutical products. Health economics is a discipline which seeks to define the costs (in the widest sense) and the benefits (also in the widest sense) of medical interventions. The purpose of this is to inform decision making and policy. It is a relatively new science and its methods are developing slowly. Health economics has grown over the last forty years as a response to the gulf between publicly-funded health care services and the demands placed upon them, ever increasing owing to advances in medical science, demographic change and heightened patient expectations. It applies economic theory to comparing the costs and consequences of alternative patterns of resource use in the field of health care.

Few doctors are trained in the aims or methods of health economics, and, to most, health economics equates with cost cutting at worst, or rationing at best. Not surprisingly many doctors have been hostile to health economics. This betokens a misunderstanding of what health economics seeks to do, which is not to save money for the Treasury but to define the most efficient means of using health care resources. This may actually increase costs, if an area of efficient health care is not currently being adequately supported.

Pharmacoeconomics is a branch of health economics that considers pharmaceutical products. It has largely been championed by the pharmaceutical industry who may see in it a defence for high prices, a support for advertising, and possibly necessary in the future for drug licensing in a world of scarce health care resources. Economic evaluations of drugs are already necessary for drug reimbursement in some countries, most notably Australia. Doctors may sometimes look on economic evaluations of drug therapy with a jaundiced eye (do any of them ever show a drug is less cost effective than one it might replace?) and may feel that the whole process is nothing more than a marketing exercise. While it is appropriate to be sceptical about many studies, the process of economic evaluation of drug therapy has the potential to improve the efficiency of prescribing. All prescribers in the future may need to understand the basics of economic evaluation of drug therapy, just as they need to be able to understand the basics of a conventional drug trial now. Doctors will need an independent source of evaluation of such economic studies, in the same way that the *Drug and Therapeutics Bulletin* or *MeReC Bulletin* operate for conventional clinical evaluations at present.

For GPs wanting to know more about pharmacoeconomics

The following section introduces the interested reader to the purpose, scope and methods of economic evaluation and provides some definitions and further explanation of terms commonly appearing in published economic evaluation studies of drugs and in pharmaceutical advertising material.

The purpose, scope and methods of economic evaluation

Economic evaluation provides a framework for comparing the costs and consequences of different drugs or health care programmes in order to assist decision making when choices have to be made between several courses of action. Economic evaluation therefore is the process of drawing up a balance sheet of costs and consequences of alternative uses of available health care resources to meet patient needs. This section attempts to provide an overview of economic evaluation to help doctors through the fog.

Origins of commonly used methods of economic evaluation

All methods of economic evaluation stem from cost-benefit analysis. Cost-benefit analysis was developed over 50 years ago to aid in public sector investment planning. In the private sector costs, prices and profits guide investment decisions. In the public sector, where services such as health care and education are often provided free at the point of consumption, prices do not reflect their true value to society.

Early applications of cost-benefit analysis were applied in the USA to flood-control programmes in the 1930s. In Britain they have been applied to transport investment projects, in particular the building of the M1 and the proposed third London airport.

Perspective of an economic evaluation

It is important to identify from whose perspective costs and consequences are being measured in an economic evaluation. They may be measured from the following viewpoints:

- the perspective of the individual patient

- the perspective of the hospital or GP

- the perspective of the NHS

- the perspective of the government

- the perspective of society as a whole.

Economic evaluations most commonly adopt the perspective of society as a whole. This is the broadest perspective, taking into account all costs and consequences of a health care programme, e.g. not only of the health implications and cost implications to the NHS of health promotion to stop people smoking, but also of the impact on sickness absence from work and government tax revenue from cigarette sales.

Economic evaluation and clinical trials

Economic evaluation covers only one aspect of the overall evaluation of preventative, diagnostic or therapeutic procedures. It should be based on clinical evaluations of health care and ideally carried out along side a clinical trial. No health care procedure can be 'cost effective' if clinical effectiveness is not first established.

Costs and consequences

In economic evaluation, it is common practice to categorize costs and consequences as follows in Box 18.1.

Box 18.1: Cost and consequences in economic evaluations

	Costs	Consequences
Direct	Overhead costs, costs of inputs into a health care programme (clinicians' time, capital equipment, drugs etc.) e.g. screening and treatment of hypertension	Physiological outcomes of a health care intervention e.g. reduction of blood pressure and reduced risk of coronary heart disease
Indirect	Costs to patients and their families of health care intervention e.g. travel costs and loss earnings due to time off work	Increased earnings from earlier return to workforce due to health care intervention
Intangible	Pain, anxiety and discomfort	Psychic value from improved health state

Source: Adapted from Drummond, 1985

Methods of economic evaluation

There are four main methods of economic evaluation:

1 Cost analysis

Considers costs alone; sometimes taking the form of cost minimization analysis, comparing the costs of different drugs, diagnostic or therapeutic procedures.

Cost minimization analysis, a type of cost analysis, is an appropriate evaluation method when the case for a clinical intervention has been established and the preventative, diagnostic or therapeutic procedures or programmes under consideration are expected to have exactly the same outcome (e.g. to prescribe a branded drug or a generic equivalent that costs half as much – the outcomes for both will be identical, and the only comparison is the cost).

2 Cost benefit analysis

Compares both the costs and consequences of different drugs, diagnostic or therapeutic procedures in money terms. It measures only those factors that can easily be assigned a monetary value. In its widest sense, this method takes a societal perspective measuring costs and benefits in monetary terms. It could be used to ask whether society would get most net benefit from spending money on building a new hospital or a new school or buying a new nuclear submarine. There are obvious and worrying outcome measurement problems with assigning £ signs to the costs and benefits of such proposals – but what other common unit of benefit other than money is there?

3 Cost effectiveness analysis

Compares both the costs and consequences of different drugs, diagnostic or therapeutic procedures. Costs are usually measured in monetary terms, consequences in some natural unit appropriate to the condition being treated. This kind of analysis might be used to compare lives saved by a highly effective but very expensive drug with those saved by a less effective but much less expensive therapy. (You might feel at first glance that the expensive drug should be used, but if you have limited resources, you may be only able to treat ten patients with the 90% effective treatment, compared to 20 patients with the 70% effective – which do you think you should use?)

4 Cost utility analysis

Compares both the costs and consequences of different drugs, diagnostic or therapeutic procedures. Costs are usually measured in monetary terms, consequences in some common denominator, such as Quality Adjusted Life Years (QALYs).

The measurement of costs

The reader may have come across a bewildering number of types of cost referred to in published economic appraisals of drugs in the literature. A few of the most commonly used costs are now defined.

Fixed and variable costs

'Fixed costs' are those such as overheads that are incurred regardless of the number of patients treated, e.g. heating, lighting and minimum staffing on a hospital ward. 'Variable costs' are those that vary directly with the level of activity, i.e. the number of patients treated, medical supplies, laundry, and some auxiliary staff on a ward. In the long run, all costs become variable because those that are fixed in the short run may be varied over time, e.g. by opening and closing wards.

Opportunity costs

Theoretically, economic evaluation should seek to value the costs of a particular health care programme in terms of the costs of the next best alternative use of resources involved, i.e. in terms of the 'opportunity cost'. For most practical purposes it is usual to use market prices of resources such as land, labour and capital. Market prices may be used to value 'direct costs' of labour and health care technology and supplies. As no market prices exist for many 'indirect costs', time waited on a waiting list for example, 'shadow prices' must be imputed. The Department of Transport has carried out considerable research into the value of time.

Average and marginal costs

Most health care policy decisions are not concerned with whether a certain service should or should not be provided, rather they are concerned with whether the service should be expanded, contracted, or remain at prevailing levels of provision. For example, a purchaser may not be willing to withdraw chiropody services, but the question is how much should be provided? What are the costs and benefits of changing the level of chiropody available? All such decisions should be based on 'marginal' costs, i.e. the difference in total cost of treating one more patient, rather than on the 'average' cost of providing the service.

Discounting

Costs of setting up a new hospital, of expanding an existing health care programme or of the long-term care of a patient, may arise over a number of years. In economic evaluation of alternative health care programmes, in order to get over the problem of differing time profiles of different health care programmes or treatments, costs are brought back to their present value by discounting streams of future costs.

Discounting offers a method of standardizing different cost time profiles so that total costs can be compared. Discounting is based on the principle that £100 today is worth more than the promise of £100 in the future, as it can be invested today at a positive rate of interest.

Sensitivity analysis

All models of health care processes, and all economic evaluation studies, involve making some assumptions where information is unavailable. The assumptions made are likely to affect the results of the study. Sensitivity analysis is the procedure of varying the assumptions made in order to see how this affects the results.

Externalities

Externalities occur where the actions of one group of people have a positive or detrimental impact on other groups of people in society. For example, public health legislation enforcing anti-pollution standards or specifying water purification standards may lead to increases in manufacturing production costs and consumer prices as well as providing health benefits.

Quality adjusted life years (QALYs)

The Quality Adjusted Life Year (QALY) is a measure of health gain developed to allow comparison between a wide range of healthcare activities. Other such measures exist, but the QALY is probably the best known. Most health care interventions either aim to extend life expectancy or improve quality of life. Just counting additional years of life given by different health care interventions does not recognize the quality of life in which those years are spent. The idea of QALYs is therefore to devise a means of adjusting additional years of life in order to reflect their quality.

QALY calculation

QALY calculation involves counting additional years of life resulting from a medical intervention and then adjusting them to reflect health-related quality of life. Measuring changes in health-related quality of life involves first describing the patient's state of health before and after the treatment and then assigning some numerical values to these states. Description of pre- and post-intervention health states in the UK has, until now, been done using Rosser's Classification of Illness, which has two dimensions, disability and distress, and 36 possible health states. The disability dimension is based on what a patient can and cannot do, e.g. able to work/unable to work, rather than on a particular medical diagnosis or prognosis.

Numerical values must then be assigned to these states based on values that are obtained from surveys of doctors and the general public. These surveys ask respondents to rank health states from best to worst and indicate by how much better or worse a health state is, relative to other health states. The responses are then standardized with the best possible health state taking the value '1', and death taking the value '0'.

It is important to note that the QALY principle is equally applicable to cases where treatments are given in order to prolong life, and to treatments which do not improve life expectancy, but do improve quality of life over years remaining.

Two examples of how QALYs are calculated follows. Both depend on a table of health states and quality of life assessments, but the health states to which they refer are briefly described. In the interests of simplicity and clarity, perioperative mortality and percentage of patients failing to gain symptomatic relief are assumed to be zero. For the same reason no discount rate is applied in these examples.

Example 1: QALY calculation for the treatment of a life-threatening condition
A patient is likely to die without treatment. With treatment he will gain an additional ten years in health state VIIB (confined to bed; mild distress or anxiety). Health state VIIB (on Rosser's Classification of Illness) has a value of 0.564. The treatment of this condition therefore yields:

10×0.564 or 5.64 QALYs.

Example 2: QALY calculation for the treatment of a non life-threatening condition
A patient is in health state VIC (confined to chair or wheelchair or able to move around in the house only with support from an assistant; moderate distress) and expected to stay in this health state for 20 years. With treatment he can move to a better health state, state IIB (slight social disability; mild distress) for these remaining 20 years. Health state VIC has a Rosser value of 0.680. Health state IIB has a Rosser value of 0.986.
The treatment provides an improvement of $0.986 - 0.680 = 0.306$ for each of the remaining 20 years.
The treatment therefore yields $20 \times 0.306 = 6.12$ QALYs.

Cost per QALY league tables

An example of a cost per QALY league table is given in Table 18.1. For each medical intervention shown, the total cost of the treatment has been divided by the number of QALYs it can provide to give a cost per QALY figure. Interventions are then ranked from most cost effective to least cost effective in terms of their cost per QALY. An intervention such as advice to stop smoking can yield a QALY at relative low cost as compared with home haemodialysis, given the data shown in Table 18.1. Although an intuitively attractive way of helping set priorities in the face of a limited budget, concerns have been raised about cost per QALY league tables and their possible use and abuse. Simple aggregation of findings from cost utility studies published in the literature into a single league table could be extremely misleading if definitions of conditions, treatment protocols, costs and quality of life measurement techniques vary between studies.

Table 18.1: Example of a cost per QALY league table

Treatment	Cost per QALY (£s,1990)
Cholesterol testing and diet therapy only (all adults aged 40–69)	220
Advice to stop smoking from GP	270
Pacemaker implantation	1100
Hip replacement	1180
Coronary artery bypass graft (left main vessel disease, severe angina)	2090
Kidney transplantation	4710
Breast cancer screening	5780
Heart transplantation	7840
Home haemodialysis	17 260
Erythropoietin treatment for anaemia in dialysis patients (10% reduction in mortality)	54 380

Source: Adapted from: Maynard, 1991

Proponents of QALYs stress their simplicity, generality and value as a common denominator in health care policy decision making. At a conceptual level they argue that QALYs allow us to quantify and make explicit difficult choices and decisions that have to be made in the face of limited health care resources. At a technical level proponents admit that QALYs are as yet in their infancy as a robust and valid policy tool and look to their future improvement.

The evolution of the QALY is demonstrated by current movement away from Rosser's Classification of Illness and valuations, perhaps the main source of criticisms of QALYs today. Lessons learned from Rosser's matrix are being put into practice in the development of the EuroQoL, based on improved health state descriptors, and health state valuations calculated from much larger and perhaps more representative surveys of public attitudes and valuations of different states of health.

QALY critics question both the concept and techniques involved in QALY calculation. At a conceptual level they question the idea of quantitatively measuring the utility, or wellbeing, that people get from different health states and the generalizability of such valuation for public policy purposes – in particular the use of average values from survey data. They question too, the assumptions of QALYs, for example, that a year of healthy life is worth the same no matter who gets it, be they young or old.

At a technical level, QALYs calculated from the widely-used Rosser Classification of Illness matrix, receive severe criticism: the descriptors are felt to be insensitive and too general, and health state valuations to be based on too small and unrepresentative a sample. A person's evaluation of different health states may depend on how the questions are asked, and this leads to potentially great variation.

Another criticism has been that QALY figures apply only over a marginal range of service provision beyond that being already provided and that this important point is not stressed enough to policy makers who may look to QALYs as a source of evidence when making resource allocation decisions.

The development of the QALY has raised more questions than it has answered. There is a continuing search for alternative and better methods of measuring health state values for the purpose of adjusting additional years of life in economic appraisal of health care services.

Further reading

Drummond M F. (1985) *Principles of Economic Appraisal in Health Care.* Oxford University Press.

Edwards R T and Bligh J. (1994) Health Economics: A Guide For GPs Through the Jargon Jungle, *Education for General Practice,* **51**: 4–8.

Edwards R T and Bligh J. (1994) Economic Evaluation of Drugs: Helping GPs to Interpret the Evidence for Themselves. *Education for General Practice,* **5**: 34–7.

Klein R. (1989) The role of health economics. *BMJ,* **299**: 275–6.

Maynard A. (1991) Developing the Healthcare Market. *Economic Journal,* **3**: 1277–86.

Mooney G. (1986) *Economics, medicine and health care.* Harvester Wheatsheaf, London.

Walley T and Edwards R T. (1993) Health Economics in Primary Care in the UK. *PharmacoEconomics,* **3**: 100–6.

Index

Milton Keynes UK
Ingram Content Group UK Ltd.
UKHW031150141024
449569UK00024B/930